1988

SO-BQY-284

G   362.6 O486
Oliver, David B.
The human factor in nursing ho

3 0301 00069446 9

The Human Factor in Nursing Home Care

ABOUT THE AUTHORS

David B. Oliver, PhD, holds the Oubri A. Poppele Chair in Gerontology and Health and Welfare Studies at Saint Paul School of Theology in Kansas City, Missouri. He has helped establish professional standards beyond state nursing home licensure requirements. In 1986, Dr. Oliver received the Outstanding Educator of the Year Award from the American College of Health Care Administrators. He is well known for his contributions to the field of aging.

Sally Tureman, MAT, is a part-time member of the faculty of the Saint Paul School of Theology, Kansas City, Missouri. She worked for three years as lay chaplain in a large nursing home and is a frequent lecturer in the field of aging. She is convenor of the Gray Panthers of Kansas City and holds membership in the Gerontological Society of America, the Kansas City Interfaith Coalition on Aging, and the Kansas City Professionals in Aging.

The Human Factor in Nursing Home Care

David B. Oliver
Sally Tureman

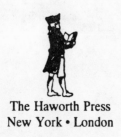

The Haworth Press
New York • London

LIBRARY
College of St. Francis
JOLIET, ILLINOIS

The Human Factor in Nursing Home Care has also been published as *Activities, Adaptation & Aging*, Volume 10, Numbers 3/4 1987/88.

© 1988 by The Haworth Press, Inc. All rights reserved. No part of this work may be reproduced or utilized in any form or by any means, electronic or mechanical, including photocopying, microfilm, and recording, or by any information storage and retrieval system, without permission in writing from the publisher. Printed in the United States of America.

The Haworth Press, Inc., 12 West 32 Street, New York, NY 10001
EUROSPAN/Haworth, 3 Henrietta Street, London WC2E 8LU England

Cover design by Anne Vernon

LIBRARY OF CONGRESS
Library of Congress Cataloging-in-Publication Data

The Human factor in nursing home care / David B. Oliver, Sally Tureman, guest editors.
    p. cm. — (Activities, adaptation & aging : v. 10, no. 3/4)
    Includes bibliographical references.
    ISBN 0-86656-715-1
    ISBN 0-86656-732-1 (pbk.)
    1. Nursing homes — Sociological aspects. 2. Nursing homes — Psychological aspects. I.
Oliver, David B. II. Tureman, Sally. III. Series.
RC952.5.A24 vol. 10, no. 3/4
[RA997]
362.6'05 s — dc19
[362.1'6]   87-36625
                                                  CIP

LIBRARY

G
362.6
0486

Dedicated to

All of the older people who have
loved us and with whom
we have been and continue
to be in love;

And most especially to
David's grandmother,
Irene McElhany Busch,
and
Sally's grandfather,
Russell Folkerth Greiner,
our first and dearest older loves;

And to the late Arthur Mohr
and the late Mattie Shaw
with whom we shared a night
in the "leper" colony.

130,708

The Human Factor in Nursing Home Care

CONTENTS

About the Authors

At first, I hated nursing homes. This was in the 1960s. My great aunt, part of the extended family that reared me, lived most of the decade in a home. In spite of the tender loving care she received there, to me the home was clearly associated with an image of a leper colony—a place in which the needs of human beings are less important than the need to keep a certain group of people in isolated circumstance. She died after eight years there—the last two years she was being turned every two hours. She died in my arms.

I took out my guilt for not visiting Aunt Pattie on the staff and others associated with the nursing home, little realizing that this same staff had become the surrogate family for my dear auntie. They had been there when she had her mini-strokes; they were there when she stopped talking; they were there at each Christmas, birthday, and at other rites of passage. They loved Aunt Pattie.

As for my part, I couldn't stand the "line up" in the hallway, the "gauntlet" which had to be overcome as I passed through the lobby nor the dayroom (activities room) in which there were no activities; the "lepers" just sort of existed in various nooks and crannies. Yet it was I that hid from them. I could not bring myself to hear their stories. I rarely approached their wheelchairs, and I did not say, "Hello in there." I could not look past the wrinkles and see the person.

My grandfather, Harry F. Busch, also died in that nursing home. He died after two months, perhaps from admission trauma. He tried to escape and fractured his skull, adding to problems caused by a stroke and other ailments. I loved him very much. He too died in my arms.

With a PhD in sociology and a specialization in gerontology, it was probably inevitable that my central focus within this interdisciplinary enterprise would be the long-term health care field. I began to teach my classes on nursing homes in the facilities themselves. I have now done this for 15 years. I have required my students (and myself) to spend many hours in wheelchairs and gerichairs, eat pureed food, sit in the "line up," and attend the various "social" events scheduled for the residents. And finally, Sally, my co-author, and I spent 24 hours as nursing home patients in a large 300-bed facility. The world of the leper colony looks very different from this perspective.

I began to see the human side of the colony only after hours upon hours of living in the midst of the lepers. They became beautiful people. They ministered to me. I am no longer afraid.

Since 1975 I have conducted over 100 seminars for long-term care administrators, top nursing staff, activity directors, and for persons who sit on various boards and regulatory agencies. I served for a short time on the Texas State Board of Licensure for Nursing Home Administrators, and for four years on the Certification Committee of the American College of Health Care Administrators working to establish criteria for professional certification which goes beyond state licensure requirements. During these years, I have learned more from those who attended the seminars, and from those on the regulatory boards, than from all the reading and research available on the subject. The field of long-term care is in a constant state of change, and there are many participants who play many different roles. I am indebted to those who have spent nearly a lifetime in this kind of health care, and I am indebted to those who could only stand it for a few days.

During the last two years I have had the opportunity to conduct ten seminars held exclusively for "entry-level" (one state calls them "lower-level") personnel; that is, seminars for nurses' aides (assistants) and housekeepers. I have perhaps learned the most from them. I owe them my special thanks.

Finally, occupying an endowed Chair (the only one of its kind in a graduate theological seminary), the Oubri A. Poppele Chair in Gerontology at Saint Paul School of Theology (in Kansas City, Missouri), has enlightened me as to the important theological and ethical issues surrounding the care and treatment of dependent adults in an institutional setting. This book couldn't have been written if it were not for the many insights of my colleagues and students at the seminary. My advanced degree in the social and behavioral sciences, by itself, was not sufficient.

David B. Oliver

When I was a young girl, my grandmothers began a foreign doll collection for me. Charming creatures the dolls were, mostly young, beautiful, or handsome, resplendently garbed in their countries' national costumes. Forty years later, after all my maturing, changes, and moves, only two are left: a scraggly bearded old Korean fisherman dressed in a simple straw cape and a white-haired Spanish dueña in somber black velvet. The young and the beautiful are gone and not missed; only the aged characters remain and are loved.

Love of older people is for me a passion, or perhaps more accurately, an addiction. As I make my way through a nursing home encountering residents, I may well fall in love with six or seven of them.

In talking to others like myself, I find our common denominator to be a family rich in close relationships with older members. I knew all of my grandparents well, and because of the family penchant for sharing stories and memories, my great-grandparents live in my mind as though I had known them. My grandfather, Russell Folkerth Greiner, to whom this book is dedicated in part, and my great-aunt, Gertrude Poteet Muir, lived into their 90s, each one active and living alone. My grandfather's many public achievements were yet overshadowed by the quality of love and acceptance which he gave to us. He will always be one of the chief loves and inspirations of my life, an anchor of security for my heart and a challenge to my mind. In her 80s, Aunt Trude apologized for not mowing the lawn. In her 90s she was still carrying food trays to the third floor of her home for her son, Bill. I spent much time with Aunt Trude in her later years coming to know and cherish her in full human dimension as opposed to the "saint" which was her reputation. Family life, therefore, has made me a confirmed lover of older people.

My first encounter with nursing homes came as a Sunday School teacher. Our church was located in an area where many old homes had been converted to "Mom and Pop" nursing facilities, a sure target for educating the children to "visiting the less fortunate." I can still taste the fear and horror of my initiation: the seemingly lifeless bodies crowded into former living and dining rooms, the vacant staring, the smells, the sense of abandonment—the leper colony. I followed through with my project out of a sense of duty, my own superficiality having defeated me before I started. Still, a spark was lit. I do not remember how she looked or anything specific that she said, but a bedridden lady talked to me about her life and the birds outside her window, somehow revealing to me the triumph of her humanness. I could not see that the humanness was all around me, but I had seen it once—the seed was planted.

Addiction to the elderly eventually led me to a year of gerontological study with my co-author, David. My final class was a directed study done in two nursing homes where I spent countless hours with every member of the drama from administrators to housekeepers. At the same time I was deeply involved with a now deceased older friend, sharing with her two attempts to "make it" at home and three different nursing home placements. Thus nourished, the earlier planted seed began to sprout and the lifeless cardboard horror became a human colony where I wanted to be.

I went to work as lay Chaplain in a 300-bed nursing home which encompassed residential through skilled care and a rehabilitation hospital. The home was located in urban midtown and was racially integrated in both residents and staff. Most of the resident population had been in service occupations—mail carriers, salespeople, apartment managers, domestics, small cafe owners, packinghouse workers, and secretaries.

I did not so much work the hours I was in the nursing home as live them. Whatever I thought I knew about older people, I was ignorant until I spent those three years in their midst. Old people can be master teachers, particularly in the arts of humor, courage, and love. Chaplain I might have been, but I learned how to play again from two who were over 100 years old, sat in the laps of old ladies at their insistence, discovered the shared joy of messy finger eating, saw faith routinely in the face of the fearsome, laughed with the terminally ill, hugged and kissed, was hugged and kissed, loved and was loved. I found families cramped by guilt and families tending to loved elders with tender devotion. I kept watch with the dying and met death in its most natural and awesome form, as friend. My work was, in essence, to establish relationships with residents and staff — to be present in all the events of living, working, and dying. I participated in care planning, staff education, and conducted 11 funerals.

From aides and housekeepers I learned wisdom and humility. With nurses, social workers, and activity directors I shared worry, frustration, joy, tears, decisions, and hours of conversation as we each sought to understand, to learn and serve better.

Co-teaching with David in the nursing homes, I have been inspired by students confronting their own ignorance and fears and been moved by their insights. In seeking answers, they have discovered, as we all must, that answers are few; it is simply being there that counts.

Before my time in the nursing home, I was, for six years, a social studies instructor teaching, in large part, contemporary primitive societies. For information, I trusted only one source — anthropologists who had lived intimately and humbly among the people they wrote about. Colin Turnbull, who spent a year with the Pygmies of the Ituri Forest and later wrote of them in *The Forest People*, was such a source. In the foreword of the book, "Vanishing Primitive Man," Turnbull makes the following statement about the nature and attitude of the anthropologist among the primitive which is perfectly translatable for me as a worker in the leper colony:

> Anthropology, by its very nature, makes no initial judgments. It observes what people do but also asks itself WHY they do it. Frequently, in this way, we come to realize that however odd something that other people do may seem to be, in effect it may be directed toward a goal that is not odd at all. . . . And the most exciting thing of all is when, instead of seeing some exotic native resplendent in robes of feathers and cowrie shells, or stark, staring naked, we begin to recognize a dim reflection of ourselves.

It is, I hope, not only love and experience that I bring to our book, but this attitude.

Sally Tureman

Preface

Many fine books and articles have been written about nursing homes in America. A careful search will find the work of those who have traced the history of long-term care from county poor farms and boarding homes to the modern day nursing home. Reforms have been advocated by many, and scandals and atrocities cited by some. Guidelines for selecting a nursing home and "how to" survive the experience have been published. Several firstperson accounts have been dramatically presented in both positive and negative terms. Books on the management of nursing homes are perhaps the most ubiquitous, followed by supplementary texts designed for preparing persons for state licensure, for social work, and for research and study in gerontology. Finally, a few anthropological studies have appeared in the literature.

There is no need to repeat what has already been done. What concerns the authors of this book is that in spite of the proliferation of research and work, which continues to be produced at an almost unbelievable pace, prevailing attitudes and images of nursing homes in America persist. The horror of living in a leper colony remains. The last place a person wants to be is in a nursing home.

Images of nursing homes can provoke all kinds of feelings and emotions. Indeed, if it were not for the negative and often painful thoughts about these places, this book would not need to be written. David recently led a two-day workshop in Las Vegas for nursing home administrators. As part of the seminar the participants were asked to go out on "the strip" (into the casinos) to interview older persons pushing coins into the "one-arm bandits."

They were instructed to first inquire of the older persons how they felt about getting older, and then how they felt about nursing homes. The answer to the first question was always very positive. "What do you mean, how do I feel? I feel great! Life couldn't be better!" The answer to the second question, however, pulled most of them away from the slot machines. They would stop gambling, get very serious looks on their faces, turn to the interviewer, and say, "Now that's a terrible thing . . . to be put in a nursing home. That's where you go to be forgotten. It's the last place in the world I want to be. I would rather be dead than live in one of those places."

We are convinced that if we asked the same questions in the church pew, the answers would be the same. There seems to be a universal negative response (at least in this country) to nursing homes.

Specific problems are subject to reform, but the basic dread of the conditions of loss and deterioration which make nursing homes necessary is not. Such dread is a sickness, and sickness cannot be reformed, it can only one cured. What the authors proclaim is their discovered truth: we have met the enemy and the enemy has cured us.

If we think of the nursing home as a leper colony, as a place where people are separated by disease (in this case, frail old age) from the rest of the population, we can begin to understand why those who live and work in such homes can feel like outcasts. They often receive much the same inhumane, unfairly discriminatory treatment that was once reserved for victims of leprosy.

Nevertheless, immersion in, not avoidance of life in the leper colony/nursing home, offers the way to healing. And it is the lepers and the leper keepers who by their humanness become the instruments of our new health.

We have chosen to act as transmitters of this reality for these healers who because of disability, position, or role are unable to be their own spokespersons. As a primary methodology, we have chosen monologue and dialogue, having found these to be the most efficacious ways of presenting our learnings.

We can share our journeys, but not more than that. Our hope is that potential travelers will be encouraged to begin their own. The humanness we found in the nursing home transformed us, and for this, we are grateful.

David B. Oliver
Sally Tureman

Acknowledgements

We thank especially all of those persons who contributed their story to ours. Without them this book could not have been written. We simply said "Hello In There," and they responded.

We wish to express our thanks to Yolanda Denise Walker, who typed our working copy into readable form, and to Cynthia Oliver who learned the mechanics of the word processor in order to assist us. We also wish to express our appreciation to Marguerite B. Oliver, whose career in Journalism helped put the finishing touches on our manuscript. And lastly, we thank The Haworth Press and Phyllis Foster for their support and encouragement as we struggled to give birth to what we feel is the real story of nursing homes in America.

Introduction

"Promise me you won't ever put me in a nursing home!" How often have we heard this plea from the lips of others or uttered it, silently, in our own hearts. The dream, of course, is to die peacefully in our chair or bed, a fitting end to a long life lived fully and independently. In a nation which worships youth and measures worth by activity, nothing so epitomizes a "failed old age" as admittance to a nursing home.

My God, I've been put in this place after all . . . How could they do it? . . . How many times did I tell them not to do it? . . . I would rather die than come here . . . And yet here I am.

I wanna go home! . . . I wanna go home! . . . Oh please, I wanna go home . . . Let me go!

I made them promise . . . And they did promise . . . Why, then, did they bring me here . . . Oh God, I wanna go home!

Why doesn't anyone hear me? It's like my body is here, but not me. Don't they understand? All I want to do is go home. If I hear one more person tell me that "Everything is going to be just fine," I think I'm going to scream!

. . . "Just leave her to us, Mrs. Brown. She will be okay in three or four days. It's always difficult for them when they first come in." . . . I think I'm going to be sick.

Maybe if I keep my eyes shut it will be easier. God, is it bright in here . . . If that intercom goes off one more time, I'm going to spit. . . . My back hurts like hell, why do they leave me sitting here in this wheelchair! Let's move! Get on with it! . . . If those wasted old farts don't stop staring at me, I'm going to tell them to go straight to hell!

Why doesn't anyone understand how I feel? First, my own

flesh and blood lied to me. They promised never to bring me to a place like this. And here I am. No one will talk with me, only at me and about me. Don't they understand how much it hurts?

I never should have let them get control of my money. Now I am powerless. At least then they were nice to me. They loved my Christmas gifts, emergency gifts, birthday gifts, love gifts, and please-come-visit-me gifts. I took care of my mother when she needed help, why can't they? . . . Women shouldn't work these days anyway. A woman's place is in the home. Now I have to have these strange women take care of me! My own kind owe me something don't they? And they know I never wanted this! . . . I wanna go home!

Why in the world do they keep saying, "you're going to like it here"? Can't they tell I hate it! And why do they say, "This is your home now, Honey." It will never, never as long as I live, be home! I wish they were in this wheelchair. I wish their back hurt as much as mine does. . . . I wish to God I wasn't here.

They've put me in a zoo! I'm a freak! I'm going to stink like the rest of them! Oh God, I'm scared! Help . . . Help . . . Please help me . . . Don't leave . . . Please don't leave . . . Take me with you . . . I want to go with you . . . I wanna go home . . . Please take me home.

A person enters the nursing home because the body, the mind, or both have declined to the point where independent living is problematical if not impossible. Losses abound. The control which once existed, enabling the individual to make adequate decisions and to carry them out alone or with reasonable assistance, has slipped from the grasp. Real and devastating are the casualties of the move to the nursing facility. Home — that chosen, personal, intimate place — has been left forever, replaced by an institution planned and populated by strangers. Only death will provide permanent exit. To enter a home is to be separated from all but a few cherished possessions. The individual has been parted from that setting, that environment, and those surroundings that declared to self and others his or her unique humanity. Simple freedoms are no more. The choice of when and what to eat is gone. Days are circumscribed by rules and routines of others' making. Stripped of the adult role, the individual experiences the loss of confidence and self-satisfaction that insured self-esteem and a sense of value and worth. Bereft as he or she feels, the seeming collusion of family and trusted caregivers in deciding the nursing home placement is experienced as abandonment. The fact that the doctor of 20 years will not be caring for the former patient in the nursing home, and that the minister of the church of years' devotion will be seen infrequently, can precipitate the sense of abandonment to an almost pathological state.

Professional caregivers are aware of the devastating nature of these losses. Yet when push comes to shove, many find it difficult to face up to the realities. Even professionals in the fields of medicine and ministry, professions which are clearly and intentionally dedicated to the caring and loving of others, sidestep uncomfortable questions and avoid issues which are sure to bring tears. In fact, both medical and religious professionals tend to withdraw from the world of nursing homes when they discover that their curative powers are perhaps no longer effective.

More than anything else, their imaginations seem to get contaminated with images of nursing homes which not only lead to negative expectations, but to attitudes which can do more harm than good. Images directly affect our expectations and our expectations directly affect our response or action. If the minister on the way to visit a person in a nursing home anticipates finding an "uncommunicative, skin and bones vegetable" who will never remember that the minister came to call, then the trip may be only out of a sense of duty. Further, there may be a desire that the visit be a short one, and worse, the potential visitor may consciously or unconsciously hope that the nursing home resident will be asleep. After all, if the person is asleep, all the caregiver will have to do is leave his or her calling card. This will not only save an uncomfortable exchange, it will cut short the time spent in the home.

The doctor is sometimes an even more pathetic case. Often he or she will not even follow patients to the nursing home, let alone visit them. Not only is the nursing home patient a threat to his or her curative powers, the number of chronic conditions may stagger the imagination and leave an otherwise confident professional in a vulnerable place. It is the rare physician who takes as much time with those at the end of their life-cycles as with those who are just beginning.

Nursing home personnel have difficulty relating to the rare visits of ministers, physicians, and family members. Often the staff becomes the surrogate family, the lovers, and the friends of the patients and the parishioners. Yet when a death occurs, no one is there to care and minister to them. No wonder the turnover is so great. Wages are low and the emotional overloads are always high.

The real caregivers are often the nurses' aides and the housekeepers. Their images can also be infected with stereotypical attitudes and leper-like myths which get in the way of humanistic caring. Yet more often than not, more tender loving care can be found between these persons and the residents in the institution, than between others. Not only do they experience greater interaction with the nursing home residents on a daily basis, they often receive love and affection from those for whom they care — love and affection which they might not otherwise receive. It is ironic, therefore, that these "entry-level" employees, in spite of the critical role they play in the nursing home, are often held suspect by the top staff, and may be fired on the spot by supervisory personnel for the slightest infraction. Professionally trained staff in and out of the nursing home have much to learn about the human qualities of the lesser trained staff: the latter often have a better understanding of what if feels like to be rejected by the larger society.

Not only are the professional caregivers frustrated and the new resident going through hell, but the adult child (usually the daughter or daughter-in-law) is likewise experiencing his or her own special agony. There are no enemies here. Most children love their aging parent(s). The decision to place Mother (or Father) in a nursing home never comes easy. Even when Mom or Dad go willingly (not wanting to be a burden to their children), the feelings of guilt and anxiety are there to stay. Sometimes those involved in the decision never fully recover from the agony of having made it.

The nursing home may be the very best place for Mom or Dad. Indeed, it may even improve his or her life-world. But it will never be home. It is time we quit playing games with the realities which await many of us at the other end of the life cycle. It is time for honesty and fair play. It is not a time for treating the elderly as if they were no longer part of the human race. We need to accept their humanness and go on from there. A nursing home does not have to be a leper colony. If there are outcasts there, it is because we see outcasts. Beauty is in the eye of the beholder. Wrinkles are the trophies of long life just as baby soft skin is the trophy of the newly born.

There are indeed no enemies here. All of us are involved: residents, family, friends, doctors, ministers, nurses' aides, social workers, housekeepers, administrators, maintenance workers, food service personnel, and others. In fact, the whole of society is held captive by the nursing home drama. Everyone suffers.

The passion which motivates the authors of this book is our conviction that the key to transforming our feelings about nursing homes is to honestly face our own humanness, learn to live with it, accept it, and even love it.

PART I: ENGAGEMENT

Chapter One

The Encounter

The images described in this chapter are real. They have been shared with us by family members, friends, volunteers, students, ministers, nurses, and even doctors. More importantly, we ourselves have experienced them. We know how they can set in motion a series of expectations which can make it very difficult to enter the nursing home.

We have written this chapter as a "firstperson" experience and will continue this style in other parts of the book. We feel the reader can follow our discussion and line of thought more easily if we make an effort to personalize the dramas played out in the nursing home. It will also facilitate the reader's identification with the themes and experiences in the book.

THE APPROACH

I am not alone in my car going to make my nursing home visit. Crowded in beside me are duty, fear, and anxiety. Reluctance grips the steering wheel. Like a child in a wagon going down a steep hill, I feel the car is going too fast for me and I long to drag my feet. Almost any excuse to turn back would do. The finality of driving into the parking lot is physically oppressive. I feel my heart constrict. Yes, constrict is the right word; my heart is not going to be big enough to hold the sights and emotions of the next hour. The next hour? Maybe my friend will be asleep so that I may leave a note or a word with the nurse and go quickly. Anything to get away and back into the normal world where I do not feel threatened by old age and deterioration.

The parking lot is filled with cars, but there is only one other besides me in the section marked "Visitors Only." I envy all those who are not here. And how disturbing it is that so many, many people are required to take care of those inside! I feel the oldness, frailness, the illness, and the boredom that require so much attention to survive and cope. Only duty and affection for my friend, Mary, propel my leaden feet toward the entrance. In my imagination it is not the name of the nursing home I see on the building, but the words, "Abandon hope all ye who enter here." This is the point of no return.

THE LOBBY

As I enter the door I realize that I can't turn back — they've seen me. Why does the entrance need to be cluttered with all this decaying humanity? If I were an architect I would never put the lobby here! Why don't they congregate in the lounge where they can watch television or look out the window? The chairs are even more comfortable there. I guess they all gather here because this is where the action is. Perhaps that's why the lounges are always empty. The natural sunlight, the televisions, and the artificial plants are pleasant, but nobody ever walks by. Nothing to watch. No one to touch. The lobby is the place to be. Here the world comes in every now and then.

I wish there were a back door. If I ever have to put my mother or father in a nursing home, I will ask the Administrator to remove all these bodies from the lobby when we come through. My dad would die if he had to see these lifeless forms in various stages of consciousness and unconsciousness. And Mom, what a scene she would make! She would demand all the way to her room that I take her back home. Maybe my brother will be stuck with that job.

Oh, no! Is that my friend Mary sitting over there with the others peering at me? I force myself to approach her and discover to my relief that it is someone else. Before I can turn away, the peering becomes a stare and holds me in stunned silence. Why does she look so desperately into my eyes? "Let me go!" I want to yell at her. Yet, my captor is not even touching me. Why did I stop? Now there are others looking my way with expectations, begging for attention. But I have learned my lesson. I adopt that "I'm in a hurry" look and continue my 100-yard dash through the lobby.

I have underestimated the power of these frail people. There is no way to avoid them. It is as if they have become a giant octopus with tentacles slapping and grasping at my body as I rush by. I turn toward faces shouting silently at me to come closer. Oh, God help me, I cannot bare to touch this slimy creature, this octopus.

Latching on, one lady stares at me through her wrinkles as if I belong to her. For a moment I see my own mother. Horrified, I realize I have nothing to say. My stomach is turning upside down as I reach across to pry her hand off my arm. Her smile disappears as I detach myself.

Even as I escape into the empty corridor, I can hear their silent cries, "Please stop . . . how about me? . . . won't you visit me? . . . I count . . . I'm somebody . . . Pl..ea..se . . . listen to my story." I walk fast and look straight ahead.

This latching-on wouldn't be so bad if these people were like my friend, Mary. She's so lovable. I now hope that she is awake. I may even stay longer if she doesn't have anything else to do. It will be good to see Mary again; she must be nearly 84 years old now. I think she is the "floor favorite"; the staff really make over her.

THE CORRIDORS

Now, past the lobby, I move quickly and purposefully to Mary's room. Corridors are strictly places of passage, aren't they? Alas, not here. Right in front of me is a human whirligig, an occupied wheelchair going round and round in slow motion. I cannot get past it. I must stop it—her. With my hand on the chair arm, I bring the circling to a halt and say, sensibly, "Maybe I could help you get where you're going."

"I'm here," she mutters, looking not at me, but at some loathed invisible object over my shoulder. "She just dumped me here. Retired, sold her house, and moved to Arizona. Put me here. Left me without anybody. Moved to Arizona." Now she is crying, her face contorted like an angry baby's, her voice filled with adult bitterness.

I squeeze past her, moving away as quickly as my cowardice will take me. What can one say to a living nightmare of hurt, rejection, and total loss of choice over where one lives? God help me, that is my own nightmare!

Two men, wheelchairs placed side-by-side. The one, attractive, smiling. Relieved at the sight, I speak. "Things are looking up," I say, "The snow is almost melted."

His eyes are intelligent and interested. He speaks eagerly. "Badda do, badda do." His good arm gestures to the outdoors. "Badda do! Badda do, badda do, badda do?" He laughs.

Oh, God, a still good mind trapped by a tongue that can utter only a nonsensical incantation instead of real words. I am horrified; he is still smiling.

The other man has been trying all the while to move, painfully scraping his one good foot on the floor and attempting, with ineffectual body thrusts, to push forward. I do not even pretend to help. Escape is my only goal.

"Badda do. Bye." Smiling and waving, the first leper calls to my back.

Only one sight in the corridor now. A woman walking slowly, using the wall rail for support. At each door she hesitates, then starts to go in. As I come close to her, I hear a furious voice from deep inside the room the confused woman has started to enter. "Get out! Get out! This is not your room! Go away! Nurse! Nurse!"

The nurse appears and takes the offender by the arm. "Mrs. Gore, this is not your room. Come with me." Together they arrive at the appointed doorway. "Look," says the nurse/teacher/parent, "I put this sign up for you yesterday. This is your room." The sign is a large paper sheet with giant magic marker printing which proclaims, "Room 106. Martha Gore's Room." The whole announcement is heavily underlined and decorated with flowers and smiley faces. Mrs. Gore's bewildered look grips my heart. Even children who do not know how to read can find their own rooms. Second childhood? Nothing so sanguine. Here the words are read, but no information is received.

Undistracted by corridor crises for a moment, I glance into rooms. In a hospital I would do this furtively, aware of the possible violation of another adult's privacy. Somehow, in this place, between the lobby and these rooms, there has been a complete loss of the sense of adulthood and privacy as realities. I look into rooms unabashedly, even with morbid eagerness. Tubes dripping life into the lifeless. A bedridden specter so ancient and frail that the sight arouses a primeval fear in my heart. Nothing could make me go into that room or approach that bed.

Onward to the nurses' station up ahead. But what is this around the desk? Wheelchairs in a row. One, two, three, four, five, six, seven of them! A lineup! The non-movers, the watchers! Next to the lobby, this must be the best place to be.

The first in line is a young man, surely no more than twenty-one. Why is one who is beginning life here with those for whom it is ending? The reason is soon obvious. His body, whether by an accident or an illness, is totally lost to use. The head lolls. He is held in the chair by elaborate strapping. Strategically placed pillows prop up rag doll arms. I cringe, unprepared for this kind of misery here. But, where else could he be cared for but in a leper colony?

Next to him is a small lady reading a paperback—a Gothic Romance. She is friendly and tells me her name is Louise. Her hands are rigid and deformed with arthritis, the turning of pages a laborious task which she has mastered—most of the time. She has hundreds of these romances and reads nothing else. "It passes the time," she tells me. But, it doesn't fill it, I think grimly.

We are interrupted by someone pulling on my coat. "Louise is in my place," the newcomer says, speaking ex cathedra. "I always sit between Jimmy and Ruth! You must move her."

Louise shrugs her shoulders and asks me to place her on Jimmy's other side. "That," I say, determined to redeem my earlier cowardly retreats, "will make you first in line!" We move. Later a nurse tells me Louise cannot straighten out anymore and must be laid in bed in the same position as she sits. Are Gothic Romances sufficient escape from that?

I'm doing better, I think, and approach Number Four boldly, grasping her wrist in order to read her name on the identification band. "Hello, Ruth."

The unfocused eyes roll toward my face. The jaw line, all bone and tautly stretched skin, juts out. "Go to hell, you goddamn Son of a Bitch," she says matter-of-factly. The words hit me like a slap and I stagger back. Totally demoralized, I move toward the nurses' station and sanctuary.

Sanctuary? In the midst of the suffering of this place, the nurses are laughing! In my own despairing mood, I feel deeply offended by their levity. How can they laugh when these poor pathetic souls surround their island desk like some treacherous sea about to engulf us all with its waves of misery? Is the indifference of laughter the only defense? As wasted as I feel, I am not really surprised that they do not notice me. Perhaps I have become invisible.

I know Mary's room number anyway. One reasonably happy encounter before I see her would surely improve our visit. I look into rooms for someone likely. Here. A lovely room showing personal touches of love and reason. A handmade bedspread. Plants on the window sill. Family pictures everywhere. The woman is seated in a wing chair obviously brought from home, a colorful throw over her legs. I enter and we smile delightedly at each other. I talk and she coos and chuckles at all of my comments. Success at last! I feel my spirits rising. From the picture laden table by her chair, I select one of a smiling young man. "And who is this?" I ask, handing the framed photo to her. "Your grandson?"

She frowns. "I was just going to ask you if you knew. Someone put all these pictures here, but I don't know any of the people in them."

The roommate lying on the other bed says, "Her memory is gone, you know. Some of her people come to see her regularly, but she doesn't know who any of them are anymore. That's her grandson Bill by the way.'' Sorrowfully, I replace the photograph and kiss the soft, smooth cheek of Bill's grandmother. She is a prisoner and so am I. I leave her cell.

THE ROOM

There it is, finally, only two more doors to go. No longer looking into the other cells, I can't wait to see Mary's pleasant, often radiant face. Thank God she is not like Bill's grandmother. Pictures on the dresser, quilt on the bed, dolls in the chair, but most important, wits still sharp. It will be a good visit. Yes, I'm glad I came.

Not bothering to knock, I barge into the room with new energy and even anticipation. Oh, my God, is it Mary? I can't move. There she stands gripping the steel post of her bed as urine dribbles to the floor from beneath her soiled gown. I freeze. What should I do? Can I get out before she sees me? Oh, my God, she's crying.

"Nurse! Nurse!" I shout down the hall. When I return to Mary she is climbing into bed, wet clothes and all. Stepping carefully around the mess on the floor and holding my breath, I lean over and kiss her on the cheek. The tears stream down her face; she says nothing.

The aide comes quickly into the room, strips the bed (Mary hardly moves), grabs a cloth and wipes her clean. I stand like a petrified tree as Mary lays there naked, waiting for a new garment.

"I'll be right back," says the aide.

"But wait, you're not finished . . .'' The words fail to convey the utter despair and embarrassment I feel for both Mary and myself. I realize I am far more concerned about my own embarrassment than Mary's. I feel helpless. I can't handle it. I want out.

A few steps further into the room and I find myself in the world of Mary's roommate. It is the first time I realize this little drama had a larger audience. I was so paralyzed by the incident, I never saw Mrs. Goldworth lying in her own bed oblivious to it all. It is as if she has shut out everyone and everything.

Recovering, I notice other things about these two worlds crowded into one. Mary's "things" are gone. No pictures, no quilt, no dolls! The cell is barren. For a minute I think I am in a hospital and all that has happened so far has been a dream. Yet it is the same room I've visited before.

"What's going on here?" I ask the aide as she finishes dressing Mary.

"What do you mean, what's going on here?"

"What's happened to this room? Where are Mary's things?" I demand to know.

"I guess you haven't been here for a while. We changed this wing two months ago to skilled care. We had Mary over in Holly Hall, but after her stroke, we moved her back here," replies the aide.

"A stroke? When did Mary have a stroke?"

"Oh, about a month ago," comes the dreaded answer. I quickly look out the window trying to hide my shame. I think it is the tone in the aide's voice, implying my negligence, that adds to my feelings of guilt. This emotional roller-coaster is going too fast.

I look back at Mary only to find her fast asleep. I am relieved. I can leave now. I pause to admire her attractive and now peaceful face. I want to reach down and smooth out the deep wrinkle between her eyes which has been such a striking characteristic for so many years. I begin to recall the day she moved from her lovely house into this restricted cell.

With George gone and four children spread from California to Maine, she was the only one left in that huge two-story, four bedroom house. In the last weeks she had shut off the heat to the unused bedrooms. I suppose her social world was already getting smaller. She lived mainly in three rooms—the family room, the breakfast room, and her bedroom. Her joy was the squirrels. She had names for all of them. One day I can remember two coming to the window as if to say, "Thank you, Mary, the bread crumbs were good today."

I can't recall just how long she lived in that big old house, but it was many years. I should have realized how difficult the move was going to be. From peaceful mornings with her pet squirrels to movement, noise, and traffic in the nursing home; from freedom and choice to rituals, routines, and regulations; from deep and meaningful privacy to living with a stranger in your bedroom; from neighbors and friends like me to few visitors at all; from trips to the grocery store, church, the pharmacy, the bank, and the doctor's office to trips down narrow corridors lined with suffering and pain.

Perhaps the stroke is not so bad. When she wakes up, she may not remember the humiliation of her incontinence.

As I walk out the door a small object on the dresser catches my eye. It is Mary's favorite figurine — a porcelain statue of two lovers tightly bound in an intimate embrace. It seems so out of place. And why hasn't it been stolen by now? And who brought it? Mary's nearest relative lives over 600 miles from here. So many questions. It might be too late for me to get the answers. I should have visited more often . . . and the aide knows it.

MEALS

Exiting Mary's room at 11:00 a.m., I am confronted by a caravan of wheelchairs. One of the drivers astride his mechanical camel waves me over. "Could you move me around this line?" he asks, "I need to get to my table." Glad of any kind of human closeness and alliance, I accept the request.

"Something special going on in here?" I ask as I wheel him triumphantly around the line and arrive first in the all-purpose room with tables.

"Lunch is at noon," he replies. "I want to be ready."

All of the "want-to-be-readies" are circling me headed toward the tables. My friend, whom I have left to assist others, calls to me in a voice of desperation. "Listen," he complains, "that woman over there is in my place. I sit on that side of the table. Get her out, will you?"

Caught up in the terrible significance of table placement, I step boldly toward the offending creature and move her before she can protest. Hastily, I slip my new friend into his chosen place feeling our mutual victory in this life and death struggle.

A nurse appears and gives me a wry look. "Meals are everything here," she says. "It's the focus of the day." As if to prove her thesis, we are accosted by a woman who cries out, "Is it lunchtime? Is it lunchtime? Nurse, push me up to the table so I can eat."

I move across the room chatting and responding to the unexpected as I am learning to do. The lunch does come finally. I await

130,908

College of St. Francis Library
Joliet, Illinois

with anticipation this high point of the day that has stimulated all these souls to early arrival and fierce competition. It is ordinary food, eaten deliberately and mechanically, seemingly without much pleasure and certainly without conversation. Some eating habits cause me to turn away in disgust. Nurses arrive with the disabled and confused. The aides begin to wield spoons like shovels, feeding those who cannot feed themselves. It soon becomes obvious that the pressure of time and number of patients takes precedence over desire and enjoyment. When I see ice cream being mixed with pureed peas on the same spoon, I leave the room.

In her nurse-pushed chair the last "luncheon guest" is arriving. She is bringing her own lunch with her, a tube with whitish liquid taped in her nostril. Her old head is down, the now too large upper dentures slipping from her mouth in a trail of saliva. She is beyond all the other needs, the special place at the table, the spoon, and the feeder—even the dentures are excess baggage.

ACTIVITIES

In the corridor again, I am greeted by a charming and friendly young woman whose pinned-on name tag states that she is the Activity Director. She recognizes a visitor and is all concern. I tell her I am here to see my friend Mary. "You are probably wondering about your friend and how she occupies her time here. Please do go down to the first floor and observe the bingo game. Everyone loves to play. And please also look in the craft room. Those folks do such wonderful work." Shame is a great leveler. With my own guilt about Mary's changed condition so fresh in my mind, I accept her lack of knowledge of Mary with total charity. After all, this is a large place; the Activity Director couldn't possibly know everyone.

On my way down, I stop on the second floor and walk by the general use room. As I look questioningly at a group gathered around a table, a passing nurse whispers in my ear, "Reality Therapy."

For the earnest teacher, reality would seem to be past presidents of the United States. "Abraham," he hints broadly, "we all remember a president named Abraham."

"I've heard of him," says one nonchalant lady, "and I've heard

College of St. B____ Library
Joliet, Illinois

of the other ones, Isaac and Jacob, too." The teacher is crushed. Reality here is obviously of a different brand than his.

A snack (or is it a reward?) of punch and cookies arrives. The nonchalant friend of Abraham, Jacob, and Isaac announces to me as she passes, "This is why I came."

On the first floor I quickly discover the Activity Director to have spoken the truth about the bingo game. All roads lead here. The mechanical caravan is moving eagerly toward "the only game in town." I reflect how I hate bingo, how every member of my family and Mary hate bingo. Will love of bingo, like cataracts, be a phenomenon of old age which appears unbidden and unpreventable? Will advanced age turn us unwittingly into enthusiasts hurrying mindlessly toward our new Mecca? Feeling depressed, I head for what I hope will be the greener pasture of crafts.

Close to the craft room door, I am accosted by a bright-eyed and vigorous lady. "Be sure and look at those fools in there," she says, leaning toward me confidentially. "We're all retired people here, you know. We've all done our share of work. You'll never catch me in there with those poor sods working for NOTHING!" She sails off in a triumph of superiority and good sense.

The craft room is spacious, cheerful, and sunny, its occupants busy and absorbed in their work. Tongue depressors, cotton balls, and old Christmas cards catch my eye. I count seven people, seven workers. The craft teacher informs me that these are indeed the regulars. If so, then today I have seen about 200 "irregulars."

THE DEPARTURE

I am adapting somewhat, no longer as shocked or appalled by what I observe. My return to the parking lot is as filled with numb acceptance as my approach was with fearful resistance. What has taken place?

I have found my beloved Mary changed by a stroke which I knew nothing about; knew nothing about because, much as I loved Mary, I hated nursing homes more, and therefore came too rarely to know what was going on with her. Now, in this new state of numb acceptance about Mary and the others I have encountered today, and equipped with better strategies for avoiding what I don't want to deal with, maybe, just maybe, I can make myself come more often.

Is this the mature adjustment to reality that the learned talk about or is my eternal soul forever twisted around the spokes of a whirligig wheelchair in the corridor, blotched in the urine of Mary's gown, dripping in whitish liquid through a nose tube, and gulping punch with a friend of Presidents Abraham, Isaac, and Jacob? God help me!

Chapter Two

The Executioners

Whether or not we are a party to a placement in a nursing home, these images and experiences in the previous chapter make us feel like executioners. We not only feel part of a living death, we fear the day when we may undertake the paperwork, orchestrate family attitudes and feelings, sort through artifacts, and sell the old homestead to pay the fee for someone to live in the nursing home. No one will know how we feel or how to help us. Except, perhaps, those who have been through it.

THE FAMILY

I arrive late at Dad's house, victim of the efficiency-robbing anxiety that dogs my steps these days. I have become a master at transforming molehills into mountains. Selecting the noon meal which I will fix for the two of us has taken me over an hour. Earlier, I had started to comb my hair only to find myself in my kitchen cleaning the coffee pot with the comb still in my hand. Indecision has made me like a piece of wood in a stream — now pushed toward the shore and a permanent stopping place, now being carried along by the water to nowhere in particular.

No such indecision haunts my brothers or my sister. Each one *knows* what should be "done about Dad." Yet the unspoken assumption is that I, the oldest daughter and the child closest to our father, will take final responsibility for what the family does. I both want that responsibility and dread it.

My older brother, Jim, recently flew in for a few days' visit on his way to an international conference. As befits the eldest son and the family's great material success, he was all reason and good sense.

"There really is no decision to make, Anne. Why you continue to torture yourself is beyond me. Dad is totally incapable of caring for himself properly. You have to be there every day to see that he is fed, that he is clean—hell, just to see that he doesn't do something crazy like burning the house down and himself with it. You can't possibly live any kind of life with your own family and take care of him, too. No way, Anne. Forget the martyrdom. The truth is, Dad would be better cared for in a nursing home by people hired to do the job 24 hours a day. But, it's your decision, Anne."

Oh, Jim, if only I had your tunnel vision! But you do not know Dad as I do. You are not "his Annie." You haven't lived so close by or been so deeply a part of his life. If it was just what was best for Dad physically, there would be no problem, but I know what he's feeling. And even if his mind is foggy, his beliefs about nursing homes are still very clear to him.

These beliefs are also clear to my sister, Gwen, who calls me long distance every Sunday and reiterates her solution to the problem in one form or another.

"Hi there, you Wonderful Person! Gosh, I realized again how right we are to keep Dad out of a nursing home after my neighbor, Mrs. Eldridge, told me about her sister's experience. The food was so bad the woman lost 20 pounds in a month. Her lovely nightgowns were stolen and the poor soul was so scared of what they might do to her that she never uttered a word of complaint! Dad, God bless him, knows all that.

"But, Anne, Jim called last week and we talked for over an hour. Of course, I told him a nursing home is out as far as I am concerned, but I do absolutely agree with him that you can't go on splitting your life between Dad and your own family. It's insane. You know, Anne, what I want to do, what I would do if I could— move Dad down here to live with me. Gosh, how I'd love to say right now—Pack Dad's things. I'm coming to get him and set you free!' But, Honey, you know my situation. George is working 14 hours a day trying to make the new furniture store a success and he's got to be able to come home to some rest and quiet and attention from me. I just couldn't give both Dad and George what they need. As for my teenagers—God knows nobody but their own parents could stand to live with them at this stage!

"What I can't understand is why you don't move Dad in with you. Your Harry is the easiest-going person in the world and just like another son to Dad. Two of your kids are in college, and as for Ginny, don't you remember how wonderful she was with Mother after her stroke? Most important, it would be so much easier on you to have Dad right there in your own home and only one household to run. But, it's your decision, Anne."

Gwen, if I thought you could receive it, I would share with you the truth that I have found struggling with myself during the long wakeful nights. That truth is that having Dad live with you or me has little or nothing to do with our husbands or our kids. I played that game with myself just as you are doing. The hard fact is that I would have no life of my own at all if Dad lived with me. He would always be there. We would have no privacy. And let me be even more honest. Whether I care for Dad in his home or mine, what does either way do to my life? I have a degree, and I had a job I loved and want to go back to. But I see the years stretching ahead and nothing in them but caring for Dad. And when Dad goes I will be beyond the point where I will be able to pick up my work again. All I can envision is going from Dad's old age to my own.

Contrast that with the perpetual youth of my younger brother, Chris. Chris fell in love with education his first day in kindergarten and has never recovered. He lives in a nearby university town where he teaches part time and pursues degrees as his enthusiasms dictate. Chris is devoted to Dad and visits every other Sunday.

"I'm really distressed, Kiddo. He's failed since I was here last. I know how you try, Anne, but it just isn't good enough. You're not trained to care for him and he shouldn't ever be alone. That nursing home near me would be perfect. It has just the right amount of small town friendliness and caring people we'd want for Dad. I could drop by every day. And really, it can't matter very much where Dad is any more, as long as one of us is nearby. But, it's your decision, Kiddo."

Sweet Brother, it does matter where Dad is. There aren't many old friends and neighbors left, but they do come to visit and he would never see them again if we moved him to your town. This is the place he chose. He intended to live and die here. To uproot Dad from his town as well as his home would be to betray him twice over.

And what about Dad and me? How would we survive such a radical amputation of our togetherness?

The secret word here, the rarely mentioned subject, is money. Dad has savings and this house. Knowing that he has these last gifts for his children has brought him happiness and self-esteem. Jim does not need or want the gifts. He has plenty of money and one grown, independent daughter. He says, very correctly, that the money and the house are there strictly for Dad's care and comfort. Chris never thinks about money, but the rest of the family want it for him to clear up the seemingly endless loans he has taken out for his schooling. Gwen needs Dad's gift. George's never-quite-successful business ventures are about to clash head-on with the college needs of two teenagers.

For me, it is this house. Harry and I love this old place and have arranged with Dad to purchase it from the estate at nominal cost. Can the gifts survive the expense of nursing home placement? The savings would go first; then the house would have to be sold to the highest bidder. I am never so tempted by what Jim calls my martyrdom as when I am considering the money and the house. Chris wouldn't say so, but he would be shocked to the depths of his impractical soul if he knew I had any other thoughts than for Dad's good care. I'm shocked myself, sometimes.

How did we get into this mess? Everything was always so clear to Dad. A devotee of statistics, he was certain he would die first, leaving Mother to the widowhood that is the lot of most married women. He prepared her well. But in spite of Dad's plans and his poor circulation, it was Mother, so seemingly indestructible, who was felled by the stroke.

I remember Gwen and I sitting in this house on the evening of what had been, we thought, our "good news" day. After a month's hospitalization, the doctor was ready to dismiss Mother to a nursing home.

"I want her to get as much therapy as possible," he had said. "I'm not saying she'll ever be able to come home—don't count on it. But, she can improve."

Gwen and I were talking and laughing with that wonderful sense of abandon that comes after release from weeks of stress, when Dad, grim and tight-lipped, appeared in the doorway.

"Do you girls think I am a hard man?" he asked solemnly.

Still in a festive mood, we answered with jokes and teasing.

Grimmer yet, Dad posed another question, "Do you believe I love your mother?"

Like naughty children, we were sobered by our father's serious-ness and assured him we knew he loved our mother.

"Then try to understand that I would rather your mother be dead than to see her in a nursing home!"

He turned and left the room. A week later Mother was dead of a second massive stroke.

When anger and bewilderment could at last penetrate my grief, I confronted Dad with his harsh statement.

"Annie, when you were a little girl, I used to go back to Ohio to visit my father's brother in a nursing home. I still suffer nightmares about that place and feel the shame of my family putting one of our own there."

"But, Dad, there are nursing homes and then there are nursing homes. They can be decent places which serve real needs. I'm sure Mother didn't share your feelings."

"Your mother is safe and at peace, Annie. I don't ever want to discuss it again."

Perhaps his conviction that Mother had escaped so harsh a fate helped allay his grief. I never brought it up a second time.

For a year or more, Dad did well. Then the circulatory problems began to affect his legs causing frequent falls. No Humpty Dumpty, he suffered bruises and bumps but never broken bones.

He wasn't so fortunate with his increasingly poor memory. I would find him seated on the stairs with his checkbook, tears streaming down his cheeks because he could no longer understand how to balance it. Forgetting that he had ordered groceries from the local store which delivered, he would call several neighbors and ask them to purchase the same things for him. I have a picture forever etched in my memory: Dad, his cheek bruised by a fall, standing bewildered by the kitchen table which held four cartons of milk, two jars of mayonnaise, and six loaves of bread. Hurt and frightened for him, I hired a woman to stay with Dad during the day.

She lasted exactly three days—breaking one of Mother's favorite plates and serving meatloaf "not fit for a dog" was all Dad could take. I went through the motions of interviewing other pleasant and seemingly competent women, but knew in my heart that my now altered father would find something done by any one of them that was "not fit for a dog."

So I altered my own life. I used my lunch hour to check on Dad and to fix a meal for us to share. I took personal days from work to do the necessary chores around his house. My own family was drafted into the battle. Harry would stop by every morning on his way to work to see that Dad had survived the night and that he ate breakfast. My daughter, Ginny, took over my evening chores and the laundry so I could come and settle Dad for the night. In spite of our efforts, Dad's needs seemed always to multiply while my attention to my job progressively diminished. The reality of caretaking won: I quit my job.

I sit in a chair gazing at my father who is napping on the sofa. The pain of love shoots through my heart. Tears of loss blind my eyes because I know that it is over. This relationship. Dad and his Annie. This is what I've wanted to hold on to, to keep alive. To the rest of the world I am Anne, full-grown, mature, and responsible. Only to Dad am I still Annie—Annie, who buys into pipe dreams; Annie, who can hold reality at bay. But, the too delicate pipe dreams have blown away and reality is not to be denied. Two myths have I abandoned today; the one, that I can give Dad adequate care, the other that I can be a caregiver at the expense of everything else in my life. Dad and I need the nursing home as much as we need each other.

Knowledge is one thing, acting on it something else. I still think in terms of escape. If only Dad had to be hospitalized; surely going from a hospital to the nursing home would be easier than going from his own home. Then the doctor would have most of the decision responsibility—and I less guilt. Pipe Dream Annie is still very much alive. Better a pipe dreamer than a destroyer of dreams.

I look again at Dad. In a few moments I will go over and awaken him. What will I say?

"Dad, Annie died this morning. It's me, Anne, the Executioner. I'm going to put you in a nursing home."

THE DOCTOR

"I have no idea why I agreed to follow Mrs. Cunningham to the nursing home. Most of my colleagues come right out and tell patients that they will have to find a different physician. I had my chance, but she seemed so sure I would come to visit her. I guess I didn't want to let her down."

"My doctor wouldn't even give it a second thought," replies the old man sitting next to me in the airplane. "He even makes house calls."

I try to avoid these revealing conversations on flights to conventions, and I rarely let it be known that I am a medical doctor. Once that's out of the bag, every Tom, Dick, and Harry wants to get a free diagnosis or share the latest operation of their nearest relative or discuss the latest scoop on a cure for this or that disease. Usually, the novel in my hands stops even the most bold soul. But this old man is different. The look in his eye is not demanding. He is kind and gracious. An aura of dignity surrounds his presence. I like him. He reminds me of my father.

"I said he even makes house calls," the man repeats. He is not being critical, only factual.

"Oh," I reply, "He does?"

"Indeed. He knows everyone in town; he's not like most of your city doctors."

"I guess he's been practicing in your community for a long time?" I inquire, unable to escape.

"A very long time. Nearly half a century. The people won't let him retire. Why, when he quits medicine folks up my way may have to move to the city."

Not wanting to defend the medical profession, I simply say, "That's too bad."

"Yes it is." He takes my signal to bring closure to the conversation with a tone of resignation.

My mind returns to Mrs. Cunningham. Why am I disappointed that I agreed to visit her in the nursing home? Why do I keep thinking that it is a waste of my time? Why does that place bother me so? It's not just her, I don't like to visit anyone there. Part of it, I think, is that just as medical students suffer from every disease they study, I see myself in every chronically ill and frail old person. The curse of my profession. But, there's more to it than that.

Out of the blue, the old man comes to life again.

"Why don't you look forward to visiting the old lady in the nursing home?"

I'd hoped our conversation was at an end. Pretending to read my book, I ignore him. But the silence begins to fill the cabin; he is waiting for my answer. Waiting . . .

Slowly I turn to him and say honestly, "I don't know."

"It's because you can't cure her. She won't respond to your curative powers. Your whole profession, your career, is threatened. When you sentence her to the nursing home, you are admitting failure. The D.R.G.s* probably don't help you much because they suggest you *can* cure her, even get her out of the hospital on time. You prescribe medicine, but the nurses call you to remind you how ineffectual you are. You give orders long distance, over the phone. You visit out of a sense of duty, not anticipation. You dread it. You *don't* look forward to it."

Silence.

More silence.

He reaches out and takes my hand tenderly, and speaks quietly, "I'm a doctor too."

I can't respond because of the sudden lump in my throat.

"It's O.K.," he says, "It's O.K."

His sense of understanding causes the first tears to appear on my face. As I lower my head in embarrassment I see an identification

---

*Diagnostic related groupings used to determine Medicare reimbursement rates.

tag on the bag beneath the seat in front of him. "Dr. Ralph Simpson, Middleburg, Michigan."

I turn toward him and say, "Dr. Simpson, my name is Charles Wingate. Please excuse my lack of composure. I guess I never realized how much this was getting to me."

"Call me Ralph. I'm the one who still makes house calls and I go to nursing homes regularly. I look forward to it," he replies.

"How do you do it? What you say is true you know. Those people in those homes are our failures."

"Once, a long time ago, I felt like a failure. I was a young man about your age. It took some time for me to realize that none of us gets out of this life alive. We all die, and many of us will need help as the time draws near. I began to mature as a doctor when I came to understand that my job is caring as much as it is curing. In a sense physicians are actually nothing more than highly educated nurses. We should leave curing to that higher power greater than ourselves. Our job is to give our best care and that may involve a brief visit in a nursing home. They love to see us you know."

"But what good does it do?" I ask, still showing my reluctance to accept his wisdom.

"We provide them hope, especially if we don't abandon them. They hang on every word. They always want private time. And we should listen carefully to what they have to say; it's the best medicine we can give." After a brief period of reflection, he adds, "Sometimes I think they do me more good than I do them. Maybe that's why I look forward to it."

Already I feel better. Mrs. Cunningham can expect a visit from me. It's not a cure she's looking for, she just wants a visit. We like each other. Simpson is right, the hope comes from my not forgetting her. To abandon her now would be to abandon my doctor's oath to do my best for my patients. I will take her the best medicine I have—myself. I'm beginning to look forward to seeing her.

"Thanks," I say, and mean it.

"Think nothing of it," Dr. Simpson replies, "My father was a doctor, too. He taught me these things about life and older people. It feels good to pass it on."

THE SOCIAL WORKER AND THE SECRETARY

"Sis, I think Mom needs to go to a nursing home!" I shout into the phone. The connection is never very good.

"What does the doctor say?" Sis shouts back.

"He told me to begin talking with the Director of Social Services here at the hospital. He said we'd better get prepared for the worst."

"Did you tell him we live out here in the country—a long way from that hospital?" she asks.

"Yes. He told me that *you* should begin checking out places nearby while I check them out here in the city. We don't have much time. He says the hospital wants to dismiss her now."

Accepting my urgency, Sis agrees, "I'll go down to Barry Hospital tomorrow. Maybe someone there can recommend a nursing home. I don't have any idea which one is best. You check out the big metropolis." The phone goes dead. My sister cares little for polite formalities.

I take the elevator down to the first floor and find the corridor marked "Hospital Offices." The receptionist guides me down two passageways to a door labeled "Social Services." I sit and wait for 42 minutes.

"Mr. Applebee can see you now," a voice calls across the room. I rise to be greeted by a tall, nice-looking gentleman dressed in a suit and tie. He takes me into his office, asks about Mom's condition, and begins rattling off the names, locations, and benefits of a number and variety of nursing homes. He explains that he is a social worker and that 30 to 40 patients are placed each month from his office.

I ask, "And have you personally visited any of these homes? Could you describe some of them to me?"

"Well, not all of them," comes the hesitant reply.

"How can you possibly help me select one then? How old are the facts you have there on paper? I want current . . . "

"Very current!" he interrupts, obviously irritated by my inquiries.

"And how can I be sure they are accurate?" I ask, gaining confidence. I will not let up.

"Go see for yourself. I will give you names and addresses so you can make appointments." The finality in his voice tells me the encounter is over as far as he is concerned. I take the list.

Revitalizing the conversation, I ask, "Is this all the help I can expect from this hospital? Don't you evaluate the homes you recommend to people like me? Which ones give quality care? What about the attitudes and feelings of the staffs? Where can Mother find a homelike atmosphere?"

His answers are so businesslike and defensive, I leave with an unresolved knot in my stomach. I hate this place. Too many germs here.

The phone is ringing. At first I think it's the alarm clock. It's Sis.

"Yesterday I visited every home within a 20-mile radius of the farm. Would you believe there are nine of them! Everyone was so nice. The secretary at the hospital was very helpful."

"Secretary?" I question, almost demanding an answer.

"Yes. Mrs. Swanson. She is the person responsible at Barry Hospital for giving out this kind of information. She told me so many things about the homes, I wanted to go see for myself. It has been quite an experience."

"Whose secretary?" I again question.

"Well, I'm not sure. She's the receptionist and general helper. She runs the switchboard, and greets visitors, but officially, she's the administrator's secretary, I think."

I'm beginning to believe no one cares about me, Sis, or Mother. Why is so little time and energy invested in such an important life-changing, life-threatening move? It appears my mother's future will be directed by a small town secretary.

THE FRIEND

The phone rings. The digital clock on the dresser shines 4:58 a.m. It's the nursing home.

"Mrs. Campbell, this is Mrs. Austin at the nursing home. I am the charge nurse on the night shift. Your friend, Mrs. Fremont, has been taken to St. Christopher's Hospital. The doctor told us to have her sent there immediately. We knew you would want to know."

"What happened?" I whisper, still trying to wake up.

"Mrs. Campbell, I'm afraid she is dying."

Before she finishes her sentence my feet are on the floor. Is this the end? Is it going to be over? Will Betty at last be free? For six years I have watched her decline toward death. Has the moment come?

It all began when Betty started forgetting where she put the keys to her car. Now I think it was because she wasn't quite sure how to drive the car anymore. At any rate, she knew things weren't right. Frightened, but realistic, she asked me to take over as her "power of attorney," and to serve as the executor of her estate and will. Less realistically, I felt honored. We had started on a treadmill that would end in Betty's being declared incompetent and I becoming her legal guardian. Little did I realize how painful these roles would be.

Betty and I were married to husbands who knew each other well. As a result we did everything together for some 30 years. We became as close in our friendship as the friendship which bound our spouses. Betty's husband died suddenly, the first to go. Then mine. As she deteriorated, I was the only one left. She had no children, no brothers, no sisters, no one. I was it.

As things got worse, Betty began to give away her possessions to strangers. She would put on several sets of clothes at one time or forget how to open her front door. She failed to bathe, could not cook or prepare a meal. On occasions she didn't even know who I was. It hurt to see her dying. It hurt even more to see her lose herself.

I know now that I waited too long to find a nursing home. She agreed to go long before the move was made, but I was afraid what others would think. I was convinced that I would be accused of washing my hands of a difficult task. I thought others would believe I was thinking of myself and not of her. But I always put her best interests first, not mine!

The nursing home was so expensive. I was informed that as guardian I would have to sell her house and belongings to secure an interest-bearing account to pay the monthly bills. The record keeping was enormous. I should have hired someone to do it, but I did it myself. As her items sold, part of me died—after all, these belongings were part of my life too. In spite of all the regulations and restrictions, it was easy for me to see how abuses could occur.

I visited her every day at the nursing home. I even took her out to dinner, often risking embarrassment because of her bizarre behavior. And now she is dying.

As I drive to the hospital I wonder why the home called *after* she had been transferred. Why didn't the doctor call me before he had Betty moved? I'm the guardian. I'm her friend. I'm her family! I've visited every day!

"Hello, my name is Mrs. Campbell," I say to the white-clad nurse at the station. "My friend, Mrs. Fremont, was brought here from the Sunshine Health Care Center. Do you know where she is?"

"Please wait right here, the doctor should be here shortly," she replies.

"But where is she?" I demand.

"We had her placed in Intensive Care, her breathing was very irregular. Do wait here."

Before I can protest further the partner of Betty's doctor walks briskly to the desk. "Good morning, I'm Dr. Mills. I believe you are Mrs. Campbell. I'm so sorry about Mrs. Fremont. I will take a look at her right now."

"May I come with you?" I ask.

"We have her in Intensive Care, so I would rather you wait here. I'll only be a minute or so," he responds.

A minute or so? He is gone nearly 15 minutes. I expect the worst. I finally see him walking slowly to the waiting area. He is preparing his speech.

"Mrs. Campbell, I'm afraid Betty is fighting for her life."

"Is it a heart attack?" I ask. "Is that why you put her in the Coronary Intensive Care Unit?" I can tell by his demeanor that my questions bother him.

"No, I think she might have pneumonia. I just thought she would be easier to monitor there."

"Is she going to die?" I am now begging for information.

"It doesn't look good. I will be by to visit her several times today. I'll let you know how she is doing as soon as we can tell more," he calmly squeezes my hand and walks down the hall.

Betty died before the next sunrise. She was a dear friend. I stood by her bedside for hours. The machines, tubes, and I waited for her to die. She only opened her eyes once. I think she recognized me, for she smiled like a lost child found by her mother. She chose to die, however, after I had gone home for a rest.

My role as guardian is nearly over. The will, the estate, the funeral, and the grave—so much remains to be done. Love is expensive. Being a guardian extracts a heavy price. I will never do it again.

THE MINISTER

She will be here any minute. Why didn't I tell her to ask her doctor what to do? I'm not a health expert. Besides, the doctor already suggested that a nursing home might be the best thing. What does she want from me? I swore when I was ordained I would never play God, but people want me to play God. They want absolution for any guilt they may feel over the decisions they must make. Sometimes I get so weary bearing the responsibility of their expectations. How do I tell her that I don't believe her mother is ready for a nursing home? It would be easier to tell her what she wants to hear.

"Reverend, I'm so glad you are free to see me. I do need help; I don't know what to do. Yesterday the doctor asked me if I wanted him to make arrangements to put mother in a nursing home. He said it was my decision. She doesn't need a lot of care, but I just don't think she would like living with us. You know Mother. What do you think?

"Have you asked her?" I inquire.

"Well . . . sort of."

"What do you mean?" I push for an explanation.

"Well, she ought to have figured it out by now. None of us living here has offered to take her in and my brother washed his hands of her a long time ago. She knows the doctor has mentioned the nursing home option. She hasn't said 'no' to it."

"Has she said 'yes' to it?" I ask.

"No, not really. I think she wants to live with us, but is afraid to ask. She doesn't want to be a burden, I suppose," the daughter speaks softly and slowly now.

"You feel guilty if you put her in a home and trapped if she comes to live with you. Is that it?" I begin to show my strategy.

"Yes! I never liked Mother very much. She always favored my brother and younger sister. They are the lucky ones. They live so far away Mother wouldn't even consider moving in with them . . . You must think I'm an evil person."

"What do you want me to do?" I back off. "How can I help?"

"Please talk to her, Reverend. Please tell her it's the best place for her to be. Tell her I love her, but I have my own life and family to tend to. Tell her she would be happier in a home than living with us." She clutches my arm as she holds back the sobs which are moments away.

Abdicating my spiritual authority, I allow myself to be used. "I will talk to her tomorrow."

Chapter Three

The Prisoners in 107A and 216A

The reason for placing our spouse, parent, friend, patient, or client in a nursing home may be their physical and mental needs or our own needs and limitations. More often, the reason is a combination of both factors.

But whatever our reasons we require self-justification; it is as if we had committed an unnatural act. We know and accept that children must move out from home and family if they are to live full lives. No such solace comforts us when an older person is moved out of their private adult world into an institution. We, and most of society, view nursing home placement as a near tragic misfortune — and the older person as a prisoner.

A prison is truly known only to its inmates — to those who live and work in it. A dedicated sociologist who commits a year to living amongst the prisoners will come out with an exceptional packet of knowledge and understanding, but that knowledge and understanding will still be limited by the reality of being a sociologist and a free person rather than a prisoner under sentence.

Nevertheless, the authors are dedicated practitioners of experiential learning. Getting ourselves and our students into "the world of nursing homes" is for us simultaneously a commitment and a teaching style. Even one day spent in a wheelchair in a nursing home can produce insights which profoundly affect both personal and professional perceptions. Time and again, with our students and ourselves, we have found that such experiences are transforming, and that without them, one remains a prisoner indeed, a prisoner of one's own prejudices and misconceptions.

The limitations of such experiences are obvious. One is not, for example, 80 years old and suffering from the effects of a broken hip or a stroke. The young and the middle-aged students and teachers will step out of their wheelchairs and the nursing home and go their way. Neither the positive nor the negative affects of old age or genuine illness will influence their observations or the challenges that confront them during the day. But, the experiential learners will have something of real value to say to themselves and to others. In many years of teaching, it has never failed to happen.

In line with the authors' philosophy, arrangements were made for the two of us to spend 24 hours in the nursing home where Sally was then Chaplain. With the nursing home's full and imaginative cooperation, the authors were admitted as patients, assigned to rooms with roommates, and passed the time just as residents would. In the morning, our students joined us in David's room where we shared our experiences and David's roommate added his comments as "the genuine article," i.e., a nursing home resident.

GETTING ADMITTED

216A

This is it. No turning back now. But, oh, how I wish I could say NO! even at this late date. I thought this was a good idea and now I find myself wanting out. All this anxiety over one day — 24 hours — how terrifying it must be for the person who imagines that this is the beginning of the end of his or her life. For some it may be the first stage of a psychological death which precedes the physical one.

What shall I take with me? Does it really matter? Normal life will cease. Why pretend?

I do worry about my underwear. They will see my underwear! None of it is really clean . . . and the holes . . . and the spots . . . Why didn't I buy some new underwear?

"Don't take your good clothes," my wife yells to me from the kitchen, "they may take something."

Surely no one would steal *my* clothes. Where in the world would Cynthia get that idea? As I pack my small bag, I stop to check my billfold. Removing the credit cards, cash, and special items, I suddenly realize that I, too, don't trust my soon-to-be caregivers.

Finally packed, I load my life into the car and head for work. At least I don't have to go directly to the nursing home.

Just my luck, no one is at the office. I must spend this time alone . . . I cannot concentrate on my "things to do" list . . . I cannot think of anyone to call . . . I keep worrying about my underwear.

I am convinced that no one going to a nursing home should spend the hours immediately preceding by themselves. The mind wanders and frets and waits impatiently for the dreaded to happen. I want someone with me. I want to talk. I want to be human.

The most difficult move, of course, is from your own home to a nursing home. Most relocations involve a move from one institution to another — usually from a hospital to a nursing home. The ultimate fear, however, is the thought of never returning to your own home. Thank God I will be back in my own bed in about 24 hours. I honestly feel like this is the only thing which is making this bearable.

Sally and I drive to the nursing home together. We share our nervousness. Our thoughts are very similar, our worst fears the same. I wonder if there is such a thing as a "nursing home syndrome" that begins with despair, fear, and a sense of utter hopelessness? We arrive at the home and before you can blink your eyes we are separated and whisked down different corridors. It happens so fast: I am suddenly alone again.

Questions, questions, questions.

"What is your name? Address? Insurance Company? Doctor? Can you care for yourself? Whom shall we notify in case something happens to you?" To say the least this is not too encouraging. "What is your diagnosis?" Even when the medical chart says it all. And so on.

I am relieved to be wheeled to my room on the second floor — 216A. My fractured hip (or so the medical chart says) gets me classified as an "intermediate care" patient. This suggests that I can do a number of things by myself and will not require continuous around-the-clock nursing care. While not required, I receive it anyway.

Surrounded by a variety of nurses, I find myself being probed and prodded. They take my blood pressure, take my temperature, weigh me, review my medical history, put me in a nursing home gown (which incidently doesn't cover anything!), have me sign some papers, and to cap it off, wrap a plastic identification (wrist) band about my arm and secure it so only a nuclear explosion could rip it off. I am stripped, signed-in, and sealed. No one even asks me my name. They leave. I sit in the middle of the room in my new portable home—my wheelchair—all alone.

I'm thinking about how it felt to be admitted (like a piece of machinery to be oiled and cleaned) when Arthur, my roommate, rolls into the room. He knows about my arrival but keeps his distance—after all, this is his home and a stranger has invaded it. He introduces me to "Ziggy," a bean-bag character who clearly serves as his surrogate friend, and shows off newly acquired skills from physical therapy as he slowly navigates about his bed without the aid of his wheelchair. His walk is unsteady, and his naked feet bleed in several places, but the slow gait and the bent body somehow stretch for the sky as he proudly demonstrates that he is not entirely like the others on this floor. I like him immediately. Instant chemistry.

107A

It seems impossible but I am both nervous and lethargic on this long-anticipated morning of our nursing home admission. I sit and stare, feeling unpredictably and unreasonably (after all, I will be home tomorrow) afraid. Genuinely afraid of I know not what. I am also incredibly lonely. I think of David and wonder if he understands what I am feeling. If he doesn't, then my loneliness is total. Is this the way a genuine "to-be-admitted" resident of a nursing home feels? If so, it is pure hell.

A scenario goes through my head. The older woman I am about to play has a daughter who is coming to escort her to the nursing home. She arrives and to her dismay, finds me just sitting here in my robe with my suitcase still unpacked. "But, Mother," she exclaims, "we've been all over this and you've agreed it's the only sensible thing to do! Why aren't you getting ready?"

The answer is—"I don't know." And I don't. The effort of making choices about what to put in my suitcase is so overwhelming that only the knowledge of David's imminent arrival drives me to action. There is a vast sense of relief when I know that my feelings of the morning have been shared. But relief is short-lived. We are moving inexorably toward the nursing home. Feeble attempts at humor are of little comfort. Though I have driven this route to work for two years with pleasure and anticipation, I now feel only a sense of strangeness and loss. As we near the entrance, I experience one last desperate surge of hope that David, tossing discipline and commitment to the wind, will drive on by and say, "Let's forget the whole thing!" Alas, he turns in and we are there. I wonder how many others have turned in here hoping for a last minute miracle that would allow them to turn around and go home.

The receptionist is a friend—or rather she is a friend of the Chaplain. Today, I am a "new admit" and greeted with papers, questions, and a wheelchair. Everyone is sickeningly cheerful and efficient while I am certain I couldn't fight my way out of a paper bag even with directions. They all know what they are doing, but I have no idea what either they or I am doing. Although I desperately want to appear normal neither my smile muscles nor my vocal cords have the strength to perform their jobs. As Chaplain, I have greeted many a new admit here in this same lobby—greeted them with my intellectual sympathy. Only today have I touched their feelings.

With the small suitcase filled with the only things I can call my own clutched in my lap, I am whisked to my room: 107, bed A against the wall. My feeling of disorientation increases as five nurses whirl around me with charts, blood pressure equipment, and a weighing chair. They are talking and laughing as if this were a normal day. The aide who is assigned to take my vital signs and other information is new, a fact which increases my now highly developed sense of insecurity. And rightly so. At first, she cannot get my blood pressure or my weight. I feel both foolish and scared. Perhaps I am no more "here" than I feel. Now garbed in my hospital gown, I answer questions, many of them centered on bowel function. I am asked if I wear dentures, which I don't, and not asked if I wear a hearing aid, which I do. Privacy is slipping away from me.

The head nurse comes in to welcome me. For the first time someone seems to be "for me." She is sympathetic with my anxieties and seems to hold out hope for a good future as we get to know each other.

"Don't hesitate to ask for anything or tell me of any problems," she asserts. "That's what I'm paid for." When she leaves, I feel several degrees more human.

Ensconced in my wheelchair, I survey my room. My roommate, Mattie, is a regular in the lineup, so I am alone. The nurse has hung up the clothes I came in, but left the rest of the putting away to me. For a moment I feel slighted, even though I am perfectly capable of doing the job and would normally want to decide where to put things myself. How quickly we develop the "helpless syndrome — I've-been-put-in-a-nursing-home-because-I-can't-take-care-of-my-self-anymore." As Chaplain, I have seen this attitude every day. Now I experience it.

Getting to the bathroom in my wheelchair proves to be hard work. I maneuver forward and backward, but there is no way I can close the door. I feel terribly exposed and vulnerable.

Back in the room, I am greeted by an excited nurse who announces that the first floor has won the King and Queen of Hearts Contest. Yesterday, as Chaplain, I knew all of the nominees well; today as an anxious new admit, I can't even remember who was nominated from the first floor.

THE AFTERNOON

216A

Arthur is about to take his afternoon nap so I will wait to get better acquainted. I take leave by telling him that I forgot to eat lunch and will therefore wheel myself down to the basement snack bar via the elevator.

"It's bad luck to go down there in a wheelchair," he warns me.

"What do you mean, bad luck?" I ask.

"It's bad luck to use a wheelchair for anything. Forty years from now you may have to use a wheelchair for real. So it's bad luck to use one now. You may shorten that 40 years to 40 days. Besides, someone will have to take you and you could very well get stranded down there. I may never see you again."

"I need to experience it for myself, Arthur. I promise I will make it back," I assure him over my shoulder as I roll out of the room.

This is quite an adventure, even fun, wheeling down the hall.

Things are getting better, I think. Once at the elevators I reach high to push the button. Anticipating the drama of being "one of them" I wait anxiously for the door to open.

"Where do you think you're going?" comes a command more than a question as the doors open wide. I turn to see three nurses staring at me with contempt. The nurses' station is directly across from the elevators. I feel like a small child that has just thrown a rock through the neighbor's picture window.

"I'm going to get a candy bar," I say sheepishly.

"What's wrong with you?" one of them inquires.

"I have a fractured hip," I reply as I hear the doors close as if they have ears of their own.

"Well then, you cannot go to the snack bar!" she says with a final tone.

I turn around and start back to the room. While others have controlled everything I have done since entering the nursing home, this is the first time I feel the full extent of what it means. It can be devastating when the interaction ceases. I have no power to influence outcomes here. How can meaning be carved out of existence if there is just one party determining the definition of situations? I want a candy bar but, I can't have it. And that is that.

Perhaps it is my body language or the look on my face which causes one of the nurses (an aide) to come out from behind the counter and offer me assistance.

"I will take you down for a candy bar," she says as she grabs my chair, spins it 180 degrees, and gracefully slides me back to the elevators.

I am speechless. I am grateful. I am surprised. Going with someone else is better than not going at all. This aide has just won my heart. I will do anything for her, and strange as it seems, I think she knows it. In fact, now that I think about it, she may have set me up. At any rate, I learn that "broken hips" don't leave the floor unescorted, and that any trip I make beyond this level will have to be carefully negotiated. This will be difficult if communication patterns continue to be primarily one-way.

The trip to the basement is not as exciting as I had hoped. The aide talks to everyone but me. I begin to feel like a non-person.

Back on the second floor I find the corridors deathly quiet. The 3 to 11 shift has assumed full authority, but the place is like a tomb. The aide wheels me all the way to 216. Arthur is awake sitting between the beds facing out into the room. I get maneuvered right next to him (also facing out into the room). The aide, unknowingly, is creating a "mini line-up" in the room. It is impossible to talk with Arthur. My neck strains as I turn it to the side in order to visit. Finally I violate these strange styles of nursing and move to where I can face Arthur directly. We begin to share stories and get to know each other.

He informs me that the 11-7 shift (the "night shift") works the least and gets paid the most. It's hard to get people to work at night, but a larger paycheck usually does the trick. I ask him how it is adjusting to different personalities on three different shifts during the course of a day.

"You have your favorites on each shift," he replies, "but I don't particularly like the people who come in at night (11:00 p.m.). They are loud, they don't always answer your light when you need assistance, and they rarely call you by your name. They keep their distance."

"Why?" I ask.

"Maybe it's because people usually die at night. It can get pretty rough and tense when a death is occurring. If it happens on the other side of the building, we don't usually get word of it until daybreak. But if it happens on this side, somewhere up and down this hall, we all know about it. I think it is particularly rough on the aides. Sometimes the new ones don't know what to do. It scares them."

"Does it bother you, Arthur?"

"No."

107A

Putting my things away increases my confidence in myself as a wheelchair driver. I'm developing some skill and my natural desire to explore new surroundings asserts itself. I practice by going down the hall to look out the window. In the parking lot, I spot David's car and think. "We could still get away!" I go into the bingo game but am overwhelmed by the large number of people. It is strange when a staff member speaks; I feel she is talking down to me. Do I sound like that as chaplain?

What better way to practice and explore than to go down to the vending machine room for a cup of coffee. The elevator is scary. I roll in quickly, but fear I cannot turn myself around in time to get off at the next floor. Two housekeeping men rescue me and deliver me to the snack bar. My gratitude overflows.

Even in the most favorable of circumstances, machines and I are not on the best of terms. I struggle to push the right buttons and collect my coffee. Alas, what do I do with it now that I have it? I need both hands to navigate my chair to the table. (Last week a resident showed me a foam cutout she places between her knees to put her cup in. The staff insisted she do it after she suffered several leg burns from coffee spilled in transit. I really didn't understand the problem then.) A nurse takes pity on me and carries my cup to a table. I am humble and grateful.

When the group at the next table goes, they leave their chairs pulled out, thereby creating an obstacle course for me. I must clear a path to pass through. Again, people are helpful on the elevator; I turn on a dime and am triumphantly facing the doors before they open.

My arms are so tired. I try to use the wall railing to assist me, but can't quite get the hang of it. A look at a fast-moving resident convinces me that footwork as well as arm work is required for decent speed.

Back in my room, I discover two teddy bears and a stack of diapers on my roommate's bed. I know and love Mattie, but wonder what a true new admit would be thinking. The aide comes in to turn Mattie's bed down; she tells me Mattie is put to bed right after dinner. Will my activities in the room bother her? Already I feel the power of a roommate over one's life. The nurse asks if I want anything. I really want a second pillow, but don't wish to appear "demanding" or "particular" so ask only for a water glass.

By four o'clock it's very quiet and I am exhausted. I lie on the bed and think I must remember to tell the nurses that the puddle of water under the toilet is not *my* puddle! I listen to Mattie crooning her hymns out in the hallway and look forward to sharing the night with this dear soul.

DINNER, EARLY EVENING

216A

Arthur says he normally doesn't eat dinner in the dining room. He claims the people who eat there are too sick.

"I eat right here in my room, David. I don't want to be around that gang!"

"I think I would like to eat in there tonight. It would be a good experience for me to see what it is like." Arthur can tell from the tone of my voice that I want him to join me.

"I'm not sure I can see what it is you might learn, but if you would like for me to come with you I will do it this one time." Arthur seems protective of me, but it is obvious he doesn't want to miss a moment we might share together — even if he has to eat with all the sick people.

As we roll into the dining room I notice very few others heading in the same direction. I expected a herd.

"Where is everyone?" I ask.

"I'm not the only one who eats in their room. Most of the people on this floor do the same thing. Actually with the new serving trays they have here, it is easier on everyone — us and them — to serve it in the room. And like I told you, it is better there." Arthur tries to defend his preference.

In the real world, mealtime is usually very special. It is a social occasion, not a nutritional event. I hurt when I think of widows and widowers when they sit down to dinner. The chair across the table is empty, the food is therefore prepared with less zeal and anticipation, and the room is silent. Why, with all these people here, do people choose to be alone? Most widows and widowers will escape, for a time, to the local cafeteria to cushion the deafening silence at home. But here, the local dining room is not a substitute.

We roll into the room. There are eight people and two visitors, counting us. The aides are beginning to bring in the trays. It is clear that each person has their turf (table and chair) already staked out. It is very quiet except for a TV which seems to be blaring out to no one — in fact, the television is turned up so loud, nobody can talk or share stories even if they wanted to. I immediately turn the volume to zero. Now no one can hear it. But nobody notices.

There is clatter, but not chatter. No conversation. No sharing. People are being fed (the "feeders") like baby robins in a nest — each sticking their mouths high in the air as an occasional spoonful of pureed food drops into the food canals.

I turn to Arthur. He is staring at me as if to say, "I told you so."

I am now very uncomfortable. I glance away to look at a beautiful mural covering the entire side of the dining room wall — it depicts a glorious Rocky Mountain scene complete with running streams, rugged snowcapped peaks, and chipmunks. Oh, how I wish I could be there. I am beginning to crave the outdoors. I can almost smell the flowers scattered about the brook winding its way through the mountains.

This scene reminds me of how bare the walls are back in the room. Surely it doesn't cost that much to have wallpaper of this sort in every room. What happens to the imagination of those who care for the needs of others?

Chicken, noodles, cauliflower, a salad, a roll (and butter) and a piece of cake, stare at me from the tray placed on the table. I am brought back to my senses.

An aide drops a towel in my lap. At first, I think how disgusting. Does she think I can't feed myself? But I soon learn that my wheelchair doesn't quite reach the required distance for easy eating. Given the length the food must travel (delicately balanced on a spoon at that), I begin to appreciate the towel. Outsiders may not realize that it is the equipment, not me, that causes the clumsy transfer from tray to mouth.

As we return to our room, I realize it has been four hours in the wheelchair. My back is very stiff and occasional cramps are felt in a number of places. I wonder if I will ever get used to it. No longer able to tolerate it, I climb into bed.

"It feels so good, Arthur. How do you stand it all day long?" I ask.

"You get used to it. They say it's part of your care to keep you up and going. You really have no choice," he replies.

My need to urinate diverts the conversation. A major difference between using a urinal bottle and standing up to do it (at least for a male), is that standing up facilitates the emptying of the bladder while sitting or lying down doesn't quite get the job done. No wonder there are so many "accidents." I knew this encounter with the bladder would eventually become a major issue. It is one of the things I worried about on the way to the home.

As I balanced the plastic bottle at a slight angle between my legs, I slowly start to pee into it. What a relief.

"Well this isn't so bad," I say across the room.

"Don't worry, you will soon be a veteran," Arthur assures me with a strain in his voice.

I look to see him pulling the rest of his body into bed. He is out of breath, but he makes it. I wait for him to get settled.

"Arthur, is it very tough being of sound mind in the midst of so many who are confused?"

"What do you mean?" he says. From the tone of his voice I can tell he is buying time. He knows exactly what I mean.

"Is it difficult to live here and not be able to share your story . . . your memories with others who might listen to them?" I clarify the question.

There is a long pause. I wait patiently and quietly.

"Sometimes I feel I would be better off crazy like the rest of them. Then I wouldn't know where I was."

107A

How do I know when to go to dinner? I wheel out into the hall to ask. The evening supervisor is upset that my bare back is showing through my gown (Is she upset about Sally, the Chaplain, or Sally, the resident?). She reties me even as I realize that certain "modesty worries" no longer matter to me.

My hunger is twofold—born of no lunch and nothing to do. So I join the wheelchair parade of "want-to-be-readies" headed toward the dining room. At the entrance, Elnora, newly returned from the hospital, is being pulled up in her wheelchair. She hollers in pain.

Nurse: "That doesn't hurt!"

Elnora: "Who's doing the feeling?"

Everyone, including the nurse, cheers and laughs at this wonderful outburst of truth.

The covered trays arrive on a wheeled cart and are left. There being no nurse in the room, we sit and wait and stare at the food that we believe to be unattainable without help. I try to imagine us, the residents, maneuvering about the room with trays carefully secured in our laps. Could we manage? Would we be strong enough to lift the trays to the table from a sitting position? Would all the liquid be spilled when we took the lids off? Would most of the residents rebel at doing a job they believe others are being paid to do for them?

I speak my thoughts to the "wellest" person at the table.

"Forget it," she states flatly. "I tried that once and there are nursing home regulations or something that forbid it."

I'm sure it makes sense, but I'm hungry.

Help comes, but I am one of the last to get my tray. I stare enviously as each one is put down and the lid removed. My menu is pink which the nurse tells me means "diabetic." I am filled with alarm. I wasn't diabetic when I came in! Do they know something I don't know? Anyway, nothing can be done about it without my doctor's order. My veteran tablemates advise me which nurse to go see. "She'll get it taken care of," they assure me.

Nothing to drink on my tray. I request only water as I have already made a scene and am afraid of being labeled "difficult." There is no packet of dressing for my salad and my tablemate cheering section insists that I demand it. They regale me with tales of "tray mistakes."

I have seen good food here daily, but tonight as a new admit, when food has taken on the role of friend and comforter, I am greeted with watery cauliflower running into pale chicken and noodles. Depressed, but too hungry to care, I even eat the orange jello, which I dislike.

I observe a genuine "new admit" cast longing glances toward us. Her own table is silent, each one absorbed in the mechanics of eating.

Mattie is in bed, gently snoring, when I return to the room. It is stiflingly hot to me, but her fat-bare old bones need two blankets for warmth. I watch the boney outline of her hip beneath the covers and the rapid, irregular rise and fall of her breathing. As her roommate, these things have already taken on a sense of importance and curious comfort. Someone is there. In her half-sleep Mattie calls out, "Mama?"

Instinctively, I reply. "It's all right, Mattie. Mama's here." Humanness creates response.

Does indifference grow with low self-esteem? The pulley string on my light is broken off and the cork board above my bed is half crumbled away, but I ask myself, "Does it matter?" Maybe with time and adjustment such things become important again.

My world has grown so small, yet I take pride in simple accomplishments. Dressing for the evening party, I begin to understand some of the residents' methods; like sitting at the open closet door to dress. It really is the most efficient way.

I am eager for the party: something to do. I am even more eager to see David: a friend, someone with whom I can really talk.

THE KING AND QUEEN OF HEARTS PARTY

The intercom breaks the silence in the hallway announcing, "Come one, come all! The coronation is about to begin! The King and Queen of Hearts will be crowned this evening. January and February birthdays will be celebrated. Cake and punch will be served to all. A special treat at this evening's Valentine Party will be a performance by an opera singer who will open the festivities."

Actually, conscription for the party began early. Aides have been enticing both the willing and the reluctant. The willing disabled have been assisted with bathrooming and dressing. The reluctant have been cajoled. Even before the announcement, the flow to the auditorium had begun.

216A

I am ushered into the auditorium and pushed to a spot among the early arrivals. As others enter, it becomes clear that the pattern is theater seating; we are being placed in rows and columns with little choice in the matter.

I stare at the door waiting anxiously for Sally to appear.

107A

I thread my way through the latecomers. Maneuvering in wheel-chair traffic taxes my newly achieved skills.

"What if David isn't there?" I worry to myself. Pausing in the doorway, I scan the room anxiously.

"He's here!" I almost shout it. He waves frantically, beckoning me to join him.

After a day as a stranger in a strange land, there are no words to describe the joy of a reunion with someone who truly knows you. No wonder the whole day of a nursing home resident can be consumed by the expectation of the arrival of a close friend or loved one.

The Party

We are both so eager to share our experiences that we find ourselves talking at the same time and laughing at the sheer pleasure of being together. We complain of common problems — sore backs and aching limbs. Living life in a wheelchair poses a whole new set of realities.

The staff person acting as master of ceremonies is obviously stalling. After a whispered message is delivered, she walks to the microphone with a distressed look.

"Due to the inclement weather, our featured entertainer cannot be with us tonight."

Putting the best face on it, she announces that we will go to the main event, the crowning of the King and Queen of Hearts.

Valentine's Day, like other holidays, provides opportunity for special events and activities in nursing homes. In this home, the nomination and election of the most popular male and female residents is a tradition and a fund-raiser for the American Heart Association. Nursing staff on each floor nominate the "floor favorites" and jars are placed in the lobby to collect votes (each penny donated represents a vote). Running as a team, the floor nominees who accumulate the most money/votes win.

It has been our observation that nurses are often reluctant to enter into this scheme because those nominated must be reasonably well and presentable — not necessarily their true favorites. Many residents are also reluctant to participate, even to the point of withdrawing their names.

We each respond in our own way to the events of the evening.

216A

As we wait for the opera singer (who never shows) I turn to the lady on my left who has been sitting in her gerichair playing with inanimate objects. "Good evening," I say, trying to start a conversation.

"Hello," she responds.

I tell her my name and she reports back that her name is "Gloria."

Thinking this is the end of the exchange, she leans over and surprises me with, "How many floors did you come from?"

"What?" I look at her intently, excited that she initiates the question.

"What floor? How far did you have to come to get here?" she repeats.

I say, "The second floor. Two."

"I came four floors," she says with a grin. She continues to tell me, with great pride, how she made it down from the fourth floor. This is indeed quite an accomplishment for persons on the fourth floor are usually mentally impaired. Before we can continue further, the start of the program interrupts our moment of sharing.

From my point of view I can hardly make it through the crowning of the King and Queen of Hearts. It is horrible. It is sickening. It is condescending. It is patronizing. The winners are shuffled up, forced to say a few words (answer some silly questions), and pushed to the back of the stage for the rest of the program where everyone can stare at them. I want to throw up.

The King is asked his year of birth, but he cannot respond clearly. So the staff member, refusing to let it be, blurts out, "Well, the record shows he was born in 1906!"

To this the old man shakes his head vigorously in protest. But guess what is going to prevail? The record. The record is going to prevail. This kind of reality-orientation is for the birds.

The birthdays are worse. Person after person is paraded up on stage, introduced, and we endlessly are asked to sing and re-sing "Happy Birthday." Even the celebrants themselves reveal their contempt for the proceedings. Some look away or down, others tolerate it by gritting their teeth, looking straight ahead.

As one lady is being brought forward, she says, "I am hard of hearing."

To this the Master of Ceremonies inquires, "Now, what is your name?"

Not hearing her, another lady (on the front row) tries to help by saying, "She said she is hard of hearing."

"Mona Nearing? I think we have the wrong person," the Master of Ceremonies retorts into the microphone.

Other staff members try to inform the MC that it is she, not the resident, who is hard of hearing. "You have the right person," one yells across the room to her.

Finally getting it, the MC walks over to the lady, introduces her by her correct name, and announces so all can hear, "We'll have to sing this one real loud because she's hard of hearing."

I want to throw up again. All this is getting acted out in front of everybody. What a disgrace. I realize that not all parties work out the way you want them. I hope and pray those conducting this one realize it is a failure.

107A

Royal trappings do not a king or queen make. Ron and Rosie are "spruced up and lookin' in their prime," but appear more rakish than regal in their askew and wobbly crowns. The Master of Ceremonies' call for a few words to their loyal subjects clashes head-on with reality.

Ron, who has had a stroke, possesses a vocabulary of one nonsense phrase and a few simple responses. But he more than makes up for the lack of words with the charm of his smile and salute. He appears to be enjoying himself until his face is in repose—then I wonder.

Rosie, on the other hand, looks glum and put-upon, wishing she were anywhere but here and anyone but a queen. Knowing her physical condition, I worry that she is in pain. David, however, puts his finger on the cause when he leans over and whispers to me, "Rosie thinks it's bullshit." Not pain, but bullshit. As if to confirm this unheard diagnosis, Rosie absolutely refuses to say anything.

But royal customs never have had much connection with reality and the two imposters are settled to reign over the evening's festivities. Imposters? Ron and Rosie are indeed special people when they are just being themselves; it is the imposition of this make-believe that robs them of their natural beauty.

The Master of Ceremonies is having a bad night. As her friend and coworker, I know that she is basically a one-on-one person (and a good one) who is uncomfortable with this type of program. It appears to be one of those occasions when a tradition has overwhelmed common sense and people are forced to act out roles which they dislike. I recall another party on the first floor. The staff who worked with those people planned it in a spontaneous expression of love for the residents and a desire simply to have fun together. And the party was blessed. Everyone looked wonderful. The food looked and tasted gourmet. The recorded music inspired one resident, who normally had trouble just walking, to perform a rousing Charleston that broke everyone up with the sheer pleasure of it.

Even tonight there are some, who if not having fun, are nevertheless more involved than bored. It is the group from the fourth floor. The fourth floor houses primarily people who have been afflicted with mental and emotional problems most of their adult lives. Many of them are regular attenders of social events — in part for the food. Tonight, I am aware of their caring side, their friendliness, and willingness to help. When a wheelchair-bound lady needs to go to the bathroom, it is a fourth floor person who, at a snail's pace, takes her. In the midst of the farce, there is humanness.

The birthday part of the program is underway. Because the weather forced cancellation of the January party, there are many to celebrate. The pattern is to call people up to the front, ask how old they are, how many brothers and sisters they had, and the number of their children. I turn to David and moan, "I would be a total flop since I'm an only child and have no children!" Even with a less grim biography, some birthday folks look depressed at being reminded of deceased siblings and absent children. We are all depressed by the endless round of "Happy Birthday to You" sung for each individual separately. I reach rock bottom when two people whom I know to be bedfast are called to the front. Celebration has been reduced to drudgery—and worse.

The cake and the punch are as welcome as manna in the desert. As a mislabeled diabetic and a genuine dieter, I greedily accept the cake when David cajoles. After all, it is compensation for what we have been through. How easily I can understand the diabetics who try to get what they shouldn't have at these parties.

Being with David has restored me and I part with him reluctantly. The long night lies ahead.

THE NIGHT, EARLY MORNING

216A

Lights will surely be turned out soon. I'm exhausted. I want to sleep. It takes energy to listen to a story even if the chapters are fascinating. What a life, Arthur. Thanks for sharing it. We are now friends.

The lights finally dim in the halls. It must be close to 10:00 p.m. Suddenly I'm aware of other lights and noises too. The dining room lights across the hall are somehow making their path to our room, and outside Arthur's window the parking lot lamps shine in all directions. I feel like an inmate with searchlights seeking my presence. In fact, there seems to be more light than before. And the sounds. They seem to emerge from the floors and walls like frogs and crickets beginning the songs of the night. There is a buzzing in the room and the TV across the hall is blaring. A moaner and groaner pierces the silent corridor two doors away.

The departing of the 3-11 shift is marked by social contagion and excitement in the hall. I can hear the cars leaving the lot below— some slowly, some loudly. The commotion seems to be the last surge of noise before the night really begins. I wonder what my new caregivers will be like. While most of my friends in the city are falling asleep in their beds, a new day is dawning in the middle of the night for my nursing home friends.

Just as I begin to doze off, the new arrivals charge into the room to check my vitals. Arthur had warned me to be prepared, but I forgot.

"This is the 'new admit,' one of them says. "He has a fractured hip and was admitted yesterday."

I realize for the first time that it is after midnight. The aides are on a different schedule than mine. To them it is tomorrow, to me it is still today.

My blood pressure and other "vitals" are checked. I'm continually referred to as the "new admit." I try to introduce myself as "David," but machinery is not supposed to talk. They simply oil and clean my parts.

They leave almost as quickly as they had entered. I return to a half-sleep until startled out of my wits by the flushing of our toilet. An aide has come into our room and is now pouring our urinals into the bowl. She has turned on the bright ceiling light, making the whole scene look like a brightly lit operating room. It is 2:00 a.m.!

I cannot get back to sleep. I can hear snoring and gagging and urinals being emptied and flushed as the aide moves down the hall. It's an eerie kind of silence. I am lonely, very lonely. I would even welcome a return visit from the aides who checked my "vitals"—at least in doing so they would hold my hand. Touch is very important—we must remember to hug those who are lonely in the night.

In the loneliness, my mind wanders and reflects on the day. I enter the nursing home and the first thing they want to know is the name of my doctor. I get to my room and the first thing they want to know is which doctor I want. No one asks me the name of my minister or my best friend or the name of the person who might just still love me! They are only interested in my external and internal vital signs. Is it that they do not know what is really vital to living?

The night turns into morning as a glorious red tint paints a pattern from the rising sun across our wall. I find myself drawn to the window, Arthur's window, all the time now. The sunrise is spectacular, but I must raise myself in order to see around the curtain which, though always pushed back, separates Arthur's turf from mine. If I was unlucky and had a roommate who refused me visual access to the outside, I would surely be depressed all the time. We build corporate office buildings with huge, full-length windows—why not nursing homes?

My back hurts more than it ever did. I came in here with a sup-posed broken hip, but now I feel like I have a broken back. After the marathon in the wheelchair and my restless evening, I seem to belong here. Even my legs and arms hurt. The wheelchair destroys my back and the bed destroys my arms and legs. The bed is so narrow my elbows hang over the sides. Quite an adjustment for someone who is used to a king-size bed.

"Well, 216A, are you ready for your whirlpool bath?" The ques-tion enters the room just in front of the aide who blurts it out as she rushes in ready for all kinds of bed and body work.

"Bath . . .?" I ask.

She is joined by her colleague and before I can figure out an excuse why I shouldn't have to go through with this (after all, you can carry things a bit too far), they have me transferred to the wheelchair and out into the corridor.

The nursing home gown covers very little, so I yell, "Cover me up!" One of the aides grabs a nearby sheet and throws it over me as we approach the whirlpool/lift, shower area.

We enter the chamber and I get centered in front of a funny-looking hydraulic lift. I very quickly figure out what is about to happen when I see the whirlpool bath behind the lift filling with water. The aides remove first my sheet and then my gown. I sit nude in front of two women. I am lifted into a cold plastic chair and securely fastened. I am nervous, naked, and I nearly panic as one of the aides pushes a button which sets the launch in motion.

At the very moment the lift reaches its highest point, but before it turns toward the waiting waters, one of the aides says, "You know, I wonder why more patients don't like this?"

With that, I yell, "What? Here I am ten feet off the ground with my head about to go through the ceiling, naked as a jaybird, with you, Young Lady, standing there looking at my privates, and you say you wonder why . . ."

Before I can finish the sentence, she hits the button and the chair turns in mid-air and moves out over the water. Before I can protest further, the machine lowers me into the tub. She only laughs as she strokes my body with soap and suds.

With my introduction to urinal bottles, whirlpool baths, and bedpans now complete, I no longer worry about my underwear. I have arrived.

Breakfast with Arthur is very special. We both know the class and Sally will soon arrive for reflections on our 24-hour experiences. We don't have much more time alone. We have shared many stories, this man and me. I love him like a father. He has given me advice, shown me his pain, and most of all, shared himself. I will never forget him.

107A

Night can evoke its own special kind of isolation and need for those who are lonely and wakeful. I recall the friendship of a late-to-sleep resident with the night security guard. I remember how the nurses took an often restless Mattie into the nurses' station and shared their midnight meal with her.

Tired as I am, I know my mind to be too active for sleep and manage to grab a magazine from the lobby just as the lights are turned out. But I am better at my new skills than my old. Preparing for bed in my wheelchair with reasonable efficiency, I have no aptitude at all for the sophisticated prose of *The New Yorker*. Even the cartoons fail to amuse. I glance over at Mattie in her bed. She is restless and mumbling to herself. We might as well be restless together, I think, as I turn off the light.

I struggle for comfort. The pillows, which I have joked about with the residents, are made of some devilish plastic material that neither stays firm nor yields and crackles in the ears when the head moves. With each restless turn in the bed, my sheets come loose from the mattress and wrinkle themselves into small pockets of torture. Wakefulness prompts a round of water drinking and bathroom trips. Humor eludes me. I think of David and selfishly hope he is awake. Every negative experience of the day returns like a burped cucumber.

"Mama, Mama?" Mattie calls out.

"I'm here, Mattie. Mama's here," I reply.

"That's good, Mama."

I recall how many times I was told today, "Your doctor will have to decide that." At home, one *chooses* whether to follow or not to follow medical advice. One adapts and compromises. In an institution, advice becomes an order and there are watchdogs to see that orders are carried out.

"Mama, Mama? Are you here, Mama?"

"Mama's here, Mattie. Mama's sleeping right beside you, Mattie. I won't leave you."

"Oh, thank you, Mama."

"Now go to sleep, Mattie."

"Yes, Mama."

The half-closed door swings open and the lights are turned on, wrenching me from the protective world of darkness. Two nurses move quickly to Mattie's bed to clean her and change her position. The noise, light, and activity daze me, but I manage to register the nurses' kindness and genuine affection for my roommate. Surely, this will quiet Mattie.

I recall what I know of Mattie—how her condition dates from the day she was discovered unconscious from escaping gas in her home. Her weakness and confusion are exceeded only by a basic sweetness of character which makes her lovable to all of us. I begin to doze at last.

"Oh, Lord! Oh, Lord! Oh, Lord!" Mattie moans.

From out of my sleepiness, I almost respond, "I'm here, Mattie." Instead I go to her side to soothe her, detour once again to the bathroom, and climb wearily back into bed. The pattern is set and goes on until dawn:

Sally dozes.

Mattie calls out.

Nurses come in.

Repeat with variations.

At 6:00 a.m. the door opens and the night supervisor tells me there has been a death on the second floor. Desperately weary resident Sally slips on her robe and becomes Chaplain again.

Standing in the presence of death, the horrors of the night begin to slip away from me. A cleaning woman who was fond of the lady joins me by the bed and we talk quietly about her and about her now grieving daughter. I place my hand on the dead woman's head and pray.

Returning to my room to dress for breakfast, I find Mattie, of course, asleep at last. I stand and look at her and laugh feebly. To myself, I whisper one of our exchanges of the night:

"Mama loves you, Mattie."

"I love you, too, Mama."

PART II: PLAYERS

Chapter Four

The Performers in the Drama

Shakespeare, in *As You Like It* (Act II, Scene III), writes:

All the world's a stage
And all the men and women are merely players
They have their exits and their entrances
And in one lifetime, each person plays many parts.

In a nursing home there are indeed many players and many parts. And while nearly all of the role players find themselves expected to play a number and variety of roles, there are certain expectations surrounding specific groups of persons within and without the nursing home setting. We have, in various ways, discussed *family members* and their struggle with nursing home placement, and we have, in brief, explored the role of *the professional* (doctor, minister, social worker, etc.) in response to the nursing home. But the lead performers deserve special attention. ·

In a sense, nurses' aides, housekeepers, and maintenance staff are at the center of all activity and life in the world of the nursing home. They must respond to *supervisors*, and while kept at a distance, they are profoundly affected by *top staff* (administration and management). Their interaction with the *resident patient*, however, is extensive. It remains a mystery why these critical roles in the drama are given so little respect and such low wages. It is unfortunate that we could collectively label them "cheap labor." Instead we will give them a label that more accurately reflects their role in the nursing home. We will call them *the caregivers*.

As we shall show, these entry-level employees (sometimes referred to as "lower-level" employees) have the greatest turnover and experience the greatest stress in the long-term care facility. They are expected to clean butts, smile when bitten, be in two places at once, not talk back, stand in awe of supervisors who have more education, and get all the work done regardless of how "short" (understaffed) the floor, wing, or unit might be. More than this, they often fall in love with those who are the recipients of their care only to grieve mightily when a resident dies. But rarely does anyone minister to their grief and few are the advocates for them when their powerless voices wish to speak. They are indeed the most important yet the most vulnerable group in the nursing home drama.

Figure 1 illustrates some of the complex relationships between the various players. *The caregivers* are highlighted, for the drama of the nursing home gets played out in their arena.

In spite of all the tender loving care, humorous moments, and day-to-day wonderful surprises which are ubiquitous in a nursing home, conflict abounds between the actors. Hostility and contempt can be felt by an aide toward a supervisor (who shows no respect or concern for the aide's well-being), and toward a family member (who could visit but does not), toward a professional (who could do so much but is never around), and toward the top administrative officer (who has so much power but is rarely seen on the floor). And while an aide may experience tension with an occasional resident, the most intense conflict erupts (covertly) with supervisors.

Caregivers, for the most part, experience direct *intimate* contact with the resident patients. In many cases they become the surrogate family of those for whom they provide care. Supervisors, on the other hand, have *limited* contact and often maintain a professional, as opposed to a personal, stance toward the residents. This in itself

PERFORMERS IN THE DRAMA

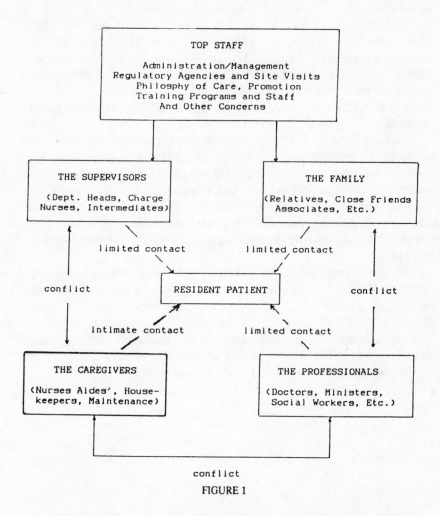

FIGURE 1

represents an area for potential conflict — particularly when it comes to deciding what is best for the resident. If the supervisor wins, the home becomes a hospital; if the aide wins, the home becomes a home.

Family members, feeling guilt or loss about their diminished role, often take out their frustration on the aide (and supervisor). If

Mom's hair is not just right or a shave is a day late, all kinds of reverberations can be felt on the floor.

Ministers arrive realizing that their presence is not only rare, but often brief. The time spent with a parishioner who was a faithful servant of the church for 55 years, but who has lost contact with the church, creates an awkward visit. Indeed, guilt for not visiting in nursing homes more often is the number one difficulty ministers have in ministry with older persons. No wonder the rare visit is not rewarding.

And then there is the family member who can't get the doctor to do more. Or perhaps the doctor is doing too much. In either case, there is not enough information exchanged or honesty shared between the professional person and the family member. And, of course, it is the resident-patient who particularly feels slighted. One-to-one, private, face-to-face discussion with a physician is all but over once the nursing home is entered. It is a major complaint of residents.

The real drama, however, is acted out between the aide and the resident. Here love and affection, rather than hate and hostility, get exchanged. A new set of intimates, the caregivers, begin to replace family members as friends and confidants. The resulting relationships can bring joy and happiness in the midst of suffering and despair. Both parties to the drama are equally affected. The caregivers, then, deserve a central place in this book.

Chapter Five

The Caregivers

After a decade of presenting educational seminars to long-term care administrators, directors of nursing services, boards, and other top organizational units, David decided that much of what he had to offer would be most useful to the "entry-level" nurses' aides and housekeepers. Indeed, the major focus of his seminars had always been patient care, and who has more direct day-to-day, hands-on contact with residents than these performers in the drama? In the past four years, he has addressed large groups of aides and house-keepers in New Mexico, Pennsylvania, West Virginia, Colorado, Kansas, and Illinois.

The majority of these seminars were held in beautiful hotels similar to the kind upper staff visit when attending an educational event to enhance their professional growth and to satisfy licensure requirements. Supervisory personnel, however, were intentionally excluded from these "entry-level only" seminars—a move which proved to be very significant. In every case, the participants felt free to express their innermost feelings of joy and frustration. Moreover, they felt important being invited (most with pay) to attend the all day session away from the nursing home.

In New Mexico (sponsored by the New Mexico Health Care Facilities Association), two seminars—one in Albuquerque and one in Alamogordo—attracted over 120 nursing assistants each, representing over half the nursing homes in the state. The course title was: "Front and Back Stage—Nursing Assistants: The Real Performers in the Drama." Part of the course description read:

> This workshop is specifically designed for those persons who have the most human contact, and therefore experience more

joy and pain, than other persons who live and work in the world of nursing homes. IT IS FOR NURSING ASSISTANTS.

The great majority of educational programs for long-term care personnel are planned for those who hold high positions in the organizational structure. This one, however, intentionally celebrates and examines the single most important role in nursing homes. Given a national attrition rate approaching three out of four failing to remain employed for a full year, it is time the critical role of nursing assistants be given special attention and understanding.

The attendees expressed a deep appreciation for being invited. They have reported a higher sense of self-esteem and have seen positive results in their daily "bed and body" work with residents. And they became David's mentors as well.

It is truly amazing to hear over 100 participants shout out, in unison and with intense feelings of emotion, "R..I..G..H..T!" to the following questions:

Do you feel like. . .

—you don't get any respect?
—you are treated like cheap labor?
—you are expected to be in two places at once?
—the floor, wing, or unit is "short" (understaffed)?
—you are treated as if you were a domestic servant, like a maid?
—you are cleaning butts all day, at work and at home?
—telling this or that family off who could visit, but who don't visit?
—no one listens to your story?
—you are powerless to be heard?
—your superiors try to remind you how *much* education *they* have, and how *little you* have?
—you are underpaid?
—crying over the loss of someone to whom you have become very attached?

Indeed, the answers to these questions and feelings are consistently, "yes, yes, and yes!" And in spite of it all, the love and affection that they receive from the residents for whom they care sustains them. In fact, some aides have openly reported that the *only* love and affection they receive is from the older persons for whom they care.

Sally, as Chaplain in a nursing home, has experienced even greater contact with aides, housekeepers, maintenance workers, and other entry-level employees. Every day for three years, she worked side-by-side with them. In times of emergency, she helped clean bottoms, took urine specimens, fed the living, and held the dying. This, of course, forged close bonds with the nursing assistants. Sally also tried to minister to their needs. A few, with whom the bonds transcended the professional alliances, became personal friends. Sally also held group sessions in the nursing home with aides and housekeepers—allowing them to release some of their frustrations and to celebrate the relationships and rewards of their work. In time, she too came to realize how critical was the role of these persons.

By listening to the stories of the caregivers and working by their sides, the authors have discovered the key to the very heart of the nursing home—a key that has unlocked the tension and the joy exchanged between these individuals and those with whom they relate.

WHO ARE THE CAREGIVERS?

"I Didn't Raise My Boy To Be A Soldier" was the title of a popular song during the First World War. The point of view was not that of a West Point graduate parent who defined "soldier" as the highest order of male aspiration, but rather that of a common run of father or mother who pictured their boy in a muddy trench dodging enemy fire. So indeed, "caregiver" is a word which can ring with the romance of high calling or suggest the pits, but it seems safe to assume that few parents raise their boys or girls to be nurses' aides.

Who, then, are the caregivers? For the most part they are persons whose education is limited and limiting as far as the job market is concerned. Older generations of aides (and housekeepers) quite naturally moved into fields of basic service as a way to earn their living. When education has been scant in quantity and poor in quality, one does those jobs which all human beings can do, but few would choose to do: "I didn't raise my girl to be a bottom cleaner."

With the War on Poverty and job training programs for the so-called disadvantaged, many young people were, and still are, trained for this essential but unsought role in society. The old baseball adage, "hit 'em where they ain't" applies here: train people who need jobs for jobs that no one is waiting in line to get.

Pay is another factor. Essential as the service might be, an employer, i.e., society, does not pay well for non-degreed basic service work (exceptions, such as the New York garbage collectors who went on strike and proved to everyone just how essential their work was to everyone, are rare and must affect a sufficiently large number of people).

A dollar or so above minimum wage is the rule here. Floor cleaners can be paid more than aides. Overtime, with or without the time-and-a-half factor, exists in some homes, but its proportional benefit must be weighed against the physical demands of basic caregiving as well as family responsibilities. Health benefits are a part of larger nursing homes, but not smaller ones. These benefits are generally well circumscribed and taking advantage of them must again be weighted — in this instance against the inherent essential demand of the job and of management that an aide be healthy and present. Aides are unionized in some homes, but it has been our experience that unions generally accomplish very little for their members. A nickel increase per hour will hardly bring cheers to the working poor, and job, illness, and vacation regulations can be so complicated and impractical as to impose a burden as much as a benefit.

Transportation is a prime factor for most Americans — for aides it is crucial. From the small, low-paying homes in the inner city to the comfortable, better paying homes in the suburbs, the problem of getting to work is foremost.

Public transportation rarely extends to the outer regions of the city or does so on a select basis which necessitates considerable walking. Departure and arrival schedules may not coincide with nursing home shift changes, while extra time on the bus and away from home may render it impractical. Weekend times and routes are chancy, sometimes impossible as far as job demands are concerned. Bad weather delays are another factor of public transportation. It must be understood that while a nursing home administrator, a head nurse, or a chaplain can be late, an aide who is crucial to the cleaning and feeding of residents cannot. In many homes if an aide is a specified number of minutes late, for whatever reason, she is automatically dismissed for the day without pay.

To an aide, then, a car can be an essential for employment. But on an aide's salary, what are the buying options? With minimum income, every dollar will already be earmarked for living expenses. More often than not, the aide will be drawn to the used car lot that proclaims "We Finance Anyone!" That lot will, in turn, be filled with trade-ins dubiously inspected and/or "guaranteed." An aide, who most needs an efficient vehicle and fuel economy, will be purchasing some more affluent person's wearing-out gas guzzler. Unless she is extraordinarily lucky, repair needs will be a constant pressure. Yet the aide, living within the tight confines of a low income, will naturally tend to put off anything that means extra expense. The brakes, which she has nurtured with care until some distant paycheck, may give out, causing an accident for which she will be simultaneously responsible and uninsured. Car insurance rates are very high in the section of town in which she lives—in other words, prohibitive, and driving without insurance is one of those risks which the working poor take in order to work at all.

Children are another factor. An aide may be married to someone of equally low-level employment, widowed, divorced, or a single parent. Day care will be too expensive, so grandmothers, mothers, aunts, and sisters will be called upon to care for younger children. Should the aide's mother become ill or die, for example, a severe crisis untempered by money alternatives will arise. Sickness in an older child may necessitate the child's staying home alone with "check-up" calls being made during the aide's break (a child's call to mother during working hours would generally be put through to an RN—not to an aide). Nervous tension and stress over children and the inevitable crises that come with them are magnified for an aide by the narrowness and precariousness of her options.

Housing problems can readily be understood by citing an incident which appeared in the newspaper. An aide living with her nine-year-old son on the second floor of a house was made homeless by a fire which occurred while she was at work. She had no insurance. In her high crime and fire area, she could not afford it. Even if she had had coverage it would not be the type that provided for temporary relief housing. Instead, she and her son were forced to move in with her mother who already had two other families crowded into her home.

An aide whose track record begins to show tardiness or absences due to illness or other emergencies is often on her way out (in a unionized home it will be when an acceptable violation can be found—and they will be looking!). Administrative and nursing supervisors justify this by reiterating the absolute necessity of aides in the caregiving of residents in the nursing home. But, since importance of role in this instance is not acknowledged with commensurate pay and respect, opposite forces seem to take an almost perverse hold on attitudes. Typically, an aide once stated, "I have a child with a heart condition. When she is ill, I need to be with her. The strangest thing is, 'they' don't even believe I have a daughter with a heart condition!"

During her years as Chaplain, Sally was called on several times to take an aide who had been injured on the floor to the Workmen's Compensation physician for examination and evaluation. On returning, she was questioned closely as to her observed opinion on the genuineness of the accident and the sincerity of the victim.

That there are aides as well as presidents of the United States who need to be viewed with suspicion is obvious. A low paying, poorly esteemed job such as that of nursing home aide will attract a reasonable share of inadequate and irresponsible people. But there is something more here—a climate of distrust and injustice created by the disparity between the aide's critical importance to the institution and the lack of respect which her role commands both professionally and personally.

Distrust and a sense of injustice are feelings often expressed by aides when they share frustrations surrounding their work role. At one seminar, David asked over 100 nursing assistants to list those things which bothered them most about their job. The top 15 frustrations mentioned in the order of their frequency are listed below:

1. My coworkers don't always do their part.
2. I have no input; no one listens to me.
3. I am looked down upon; I get no respect.
4. I am overworked, and chewed out when behind.
5. I am expected to be in two places at once.
6. Educational differences are thrown in my face.
7. Family members who feel guilty take it out on me.
8. I get no respect from the administration.
9. I get frustrated by "demanding" families.
10. I get mad at family members who don't visit.
11. I get upset with me, I lose my temper too often.
12. I don't have enough time to spend with residents.
13. Some residents are overly demanding.
14. I get no respect from families.
15. I am underpaid with very little or no benefits.

Lack of respect from coworkers, administration, families, and even residents is a recurring theme. And demands from supervisors, family members, and residents often put the aide in a no-win situation.

STORIES OF FRUSTRATION

Gracie was vulnerable, her days as aide in the home probably numbered—just waiting for the right incident, the "final straw" as her supervisor would see it.

Gracie had grown close to an aggressive and demanding resident. Vera was terminally ill and had severe breathing problems, a physical stress that often makes people "difficult" from a nursing standpoint. "You've got to find out what's in a person before you can reach them," Gracie said.

Sally was experiencing Vera in a similar way. Vera would make a request of Sally, and at the same time, present a check donation for the Chaplain's Fund. This occurred before Sally could accept or reject the request, and it was pressed on her in spite of protests. Vera was a person who had always used money to influence people and to pay for services rendered. She saw no reason to change now.

For Sally, as Chaplain, Vera's style was an annoyance; for Gracie, as aide, it was dangerous. In making a request of Gracie which went beyond her aide duties, Vera tucked a folded check behind Gracie's pinned-on plastic name tag. Regulations in the home forbid aides accepting money gifts from residents. Gracie turned the check over to her supervisor without looking at it, but later stated, "I don't think my supervisor ever felt the same about me after that—she didn't trust me."

On the "last straw" day, Gracie was beset with trouble. She hadn't eaten breakfast and had put off taking her blood pressure medicine until her break when she could take it with food as prescribed. She had heard there would be no overtime for the next two weeks, a loss of opportunity for money she needed. Her caseload was mostly heavy-care persons requiring much time and superior stamina, neither of which she had that day. Gracie's request to an LPN for help with a particularly difficult patient was turned down, causing her a few brief tears of hurt and frustration.

On a day such as this we have observed that many aides weep quietly and/or talk to themselves as they work. When Gracie, driven by no breakfast, a heavy work load, and lack of help said, "This damn place is going to hell," she was, quite literally, talking to herself. Unfortunately, her supervisor overheard the remark and insisted Gracie apologize to the patient she had sworn in front of—a request which struck Gracie as absurd since she had been talking to herself. Never the twain shall meet.

As Gracie left for her break—for food and medicine at last—she was followed by her supervisor who announced that she was referring Gracie for termination for using "abusive language in front of a patient." A perfect ending for a classic bad day.

Gracie decided against contesting her firing—"What would I gain if I came back?" Once a supervisor is antagonistic, merely getting the old job back may seem an effort in futility. Aides will sometimes use the arbitration process when they know someone has lied about them and/or unemployment compensation is at stake.

Gracie did have some final comments:

> I'm a human being, too. I get tired. I'm only one person and I felt like I was going to have a stroke. I went down to apply for food stamps the other day: I shouldn't feel such pride, but it

was hard to ask for that kind of help. I worry about the patients who loved me, but God saw this coming and will send someone to take my place.

A week or so after Gracie's firing, Vera was taken to the hospital where she died. The floor supervisor called Sally to see if she knew where Vera kept some important papers. Sally said "No," but she would call Gracie. Gracie knew; aides always know.

Aides in many homes complain of being treated dishonestly or patronizingly by supervisors. Lillie, speaking of herself and two other aides being transferred to another floor:

> Why do they treat us like children? If they'd said we were hanging around together and talking too much — well, that was true. But, instead, they say, "We're upgrading the floor."

Several aides comment on heavy care:

> Having such a heavy load wouldn't be so bad if it was only for a day or two, but you know it's going to go on and on, day after day.

> I felt so guilty yesterday because of the way I fed Anna. I had five hard feeders and I only had 15 minutes left when I got to her. It takes her five minutes to chew each bite, so I just had to give up with only part of her food eaten.

> The worst part when I go home at night isn't that I'm so tired. It's knowing I've been too rushed to really give the kind of care and attention to people that they should have. It's so frustrating you want to quit and try another home to see if it's any better.

An aide on LPNs:

> I don't like LPNs . . . they think they're boss. They think they can run over the top of you . . . tell you what you're doing wrong . . . yet they make no wrong. They're the most perfect people you ever met. But I've found out they make mistakes just like you would do. You try to help them out in their work and then they fault you for it. Only one LPN I've ever worked

with has really gotten down and done the work . . . the same kind of work I was doing. This LPN would help get people up . . . She would work with the aides and help us get it done. But generally, even when we were shorthanded, the LPNs wouldn't help you do anything. If you ask for help, most LPNs look at you like you were crazy.

An older aide on LPNs:

One home where I worked, my supervisor told me they would help me become an LPN . . . pay some of my tuition and give me time to go to school. But I said no because I didn't want to become like that . . . sitting behind a desk, forgetting where I'd come from, not caring about the residents like I do now and feeling superior to the aides. It would have meant more money which I need, but I have to live with myself.

Two aides on residents:

It's funny about difficult residents. The mean ones don't bother me at all . . . I really enjoy them. What I can't stand are the whiners. Nothing's ever right for Mrs. Jensen. Her husband didn't do right by her and she's full of complaints about her sister who she lived with after she became a widow. I think her husband and sister may have died just to get away from Mrs. Jensen. Now, *I* can't do anything right for her. No matter how gentle I try to be I'm "too rough" according to her. She can't sleep at night because it's too light or too dark in the room, too noisy or too quiet. The food's too hot or too cold, too salty or too bland. Her bowels either don't move at all or she has diarrhea. I've tried kindness, humor, prayer, and ignoring her. Nothing helps. Now I just grit my teeth and feel "kin" to her children who rarely come to see her.

Mr. Howard was the worst . . . a great big, mean man who had had a stoke. He was so mean and angry, and he couldn't hit anymore. I guess the only way he could get it out was to bite. The worst part was, he didn't like women taking care of him and a male aide wasn't always handy. They did try to assign a man to him if they could. It was hard work trying to take care of Mr. Howard and watch out for yourself at the same time. Karen got fired because of him. One day when she wasn't watching or being too careful about what she said to him, he bit her hard. She was so surprised and in pain that she bit him back. It was really terrible and everyone was so upset. It's never right to hurt a resident, but we all felt sorry for Karen . . . anyone can be driven to do something they wouldn't normally do. All the aides knew it might have been one of us.

Aides on families:

A man came once to give a talk to us nurses about residents' families. He said some of them feel so guilty about putting their loved one in a nursing home that they take it out on the staff. I knew just what he meant because of Mrs. Morton's daughters. Those "girls" were forever talking about how they wished they could care for their mother in their own homes, but couldn't for this or that reason. You know how it is when people just talk too much about a thing? They really didn't want to take care of her, they just felt guilty about it. And complain! I remember the time Mrs. Morton had a weak spell and fell getting off the toilet. No one could have known it was going to happen. The daughters almost called in the FBI and we all had to go down to the Director's office and explain and defend ourselves. Mrs. Morton wasn't hurt bad, but those girls were out for blood.

In the smaller nursing home where I work in the evening, it would have been different. Mrs. Barnes, who is the owner and director, would have told the family to find another place if they didn't approve of the care. She always says, "I pick my aides myself and train them . . . so I back their work." Sometimes Mrs. B. will question an aide in private about what she has done, but she always stands up for us in front of the family.

I had to put my aunt in a nursing home last summer and it really taught me a lesson. Lots of things aren't right . . . you find your loved one wet or the food tray's there but no one has set it up so they can eat . . . they are still lying in bed or they have been sitting up too long . . . they say no one comes when they call or nurses are mean to them. And you want to blame someone because you're upset and the first person that comes to mind is the aide. It must be her fault. I'm an aide myself— and that's just the way I felt.

With all the frustrations that confront entry-level personnel in the world of the nursing home, it is worth asking what keeps them coming to work each day. What is the source of their job satisfaction, their morale?

The aides who reported the frustrations listed earlier were also asked to list what gave them the most satisfaction in their work. The top 15 satisfactions mentioned in the order of their frequency were:

1. The joy of helping and caring for the residents.
2. The appreciation I receive from those I care for.
3. I enjoy my work with older persons.
4. The smiles I get when I get on the floor.
5. Having residents tell me they love me.
6. Being missed by the residents when gone from work.
7. Getting real hugs or real tears of happiness.
8. Getting paid.
9. Being thanked by a coworker or a supervisor.
10. Listening to the stories of the residents.
11. Residents remembering good times we have shared.
12. Being there for residents who don't have families.
13. I like older persons more than younger persons.
14. It teaches you to really care and love someone.
15. Seeing a resident go home.

Clearly the theme here is the joy and appreciation aides experience and receive from the residents. Human relationships, more than "professional" ones, seem to engage aides in a drama of living which few other occupations can offer.

STORIES OF SATISFACTION

David once asked a group of nurses' aides to write down some of their "lived moments," special times they would never forget in their nursing home work. Below are three typical stories celebrating the special relationships which develop between residents and their caregivers.

Mabel

Up until her death, she was constantly reminding herself who she was. It seemed she did this so life would not leave her. For instance, when she was up, she would start each day by saying:

"My name is Mabel.

I live in a graystone house.

I belong to the Methodist Church.

I have eight sons.

My husband works for the railroad.

Now I have to catch the school bus for school."

She would then lean over and kiss me. She did this every morning with me for two years! Then on the morning of the day she died, she didn't go through her daily talking routine. She just kissed me and said, "I love you."

Pearl

When I was feeling bad one time, I went into the room of a woman who never said much. I sat down and cried—hard, for a very long time. The woman slowly turned over in her bed and said: "Dar-ling, what is wrong? Why are you crying?" I shared my hurt, and she sat with me, talked with me, and comforted me. Then she gave me a big hug. I felt needed and very, very good.

Virginia

Every time she eats, she has diarrhea. Nothing stays with her, it all comes out. It makes me feel so bad to watch her do that. I don't like to sit with her and talk, but she says it makes her feel safe to have someone right there with her. I think she is afraid to die. And she wants me to be there at her side when she does. One day she said to me, "At least someone cares and that person is you." That made me feel proud. She is

lonely and doesn't have any relatives. She feels totally unloved, but she knows I love her, and I do.

Stories like this are duplicated over and over, everyday, in nursing homes. The love and affection which get exchanged are more
powerful than life itself. The aides become surrogate confidants and
close friends to their charges.

Exchanging care, concern, and affection is not without cost. Entry-level staff can fall in love with residents, but they pay a price.
Eventually the resident dies, and grieving patterns on the floor tell
who was doing the loving.

In a nursing home, lasting relationships are not common. Grieving and suffering are ubiquitous when the bonds of friendship are
broken by death. In fact, it is not unusual for some staff to begin
keeping distance between themselves and residents. They may do
this not for "professional" reasons, but rather because they have
learned that if they become too attached, they will grieve. Worse,
no one will be there to minister to their needs unless there is a
Chaplain in the home, and that is a rarity.

Aides have particularly been hurt when they show up for work
on, say, the 3 - 11 shift, and find a different person in the bed of a
beloved individual who had become an intimate part of their lives.
Yet no one notified them of the early morning death. No one called.
Family was notified, but the "real family" was not.

Nothing is more painful than grief. Nothing. We feel anger,
heartbreak, and a sense of abandonment. Grief keeps us up at night.
It makes us sigh. It makes us cry. The constant image of the deceased haunts and tortures us.

Another "lived moment" story illustrates the reality of grief reactions and the inevitable encounter with it. An aide writes:

I was at work one day when a bathroom emergency light began
buzzing. I went to see who it was and found Mrs. Williams.
She said "Oh, I am so glad to see you." I told her, "Why
thank you." I proceeded to help her off the toilet, and cleaned
her up. After I was finished, she said, "Thank you." I told her
she was welcome. Then as I started to turn her around to sit in
her wheelchair, she died in my arms. She had a heart attack. I

took it very hard and cried all evening. I guess one of the reasons it was so hard was because it reminded me of my mother who had died in my arms nearly a year ago.

Living and working in an environment filled with the drama of life and death on a daily basis cannot be matched in many other occupational settings. The deaths would not be so bad if it were not for the fact that the caregivers care so much.

Friendships established between residents and entry-level personnel can indeed lead to family-like relationships. The transition, however, is not made without frustration and struggle. In order to make new friends it is imperative that some level of trust be established, and established at a time when many residents don't trust anyone. After all, to be uprooted from your home of 60 or more years and placed in a nursing home, your last choice of residence, is reason enough to develop a good case of paranoia. In fact, most nursing homes can tell you at least one story about a family who brought their relative to the home, telling them that they were just going for a ride. Worse, some have been known to drop off their relative at the door and let the nursing home staff take it from there. Fortunately these are rare cases, but they do occur.

Suspicion, anger, disappointment, and depression can easily become barriers to the formation of trusting relationships, whether personal or professional. Aides and housekeepers must remain patient and hopeful that the new resident will "adjust" to their new social world. The stories below, written and shared by nurses' aides, reflect the reluctance and hope surrounding the give and take which gets played out in every nursing home.

Mr. Sanchez

A week ago water was turned off in the city because of a busted water line. Mr. Sanchez is a man whose hobby at his age is sitting on the toilet. Well, the toilet wouldn't flush, and he accused us of turning off the water purposely. It was not until I had shown him three other non-flushing toilets that he was satisfied. Thank God for His (God's) patience. The man nearly drove me up the wall.

Robert

He had cancer of the stomach and we all knew he was going to die. He knew he was going to die. To me it meant much because for months I had seen him suffer with excruciating pain no matter what was given to him. He was always bitter and angry, and I didn't blame him. Most times he was very quiet and seemed so lonely. He rarely had a positive response when I tried to show him that I cared. But it made me feel like I did something to show him I cared when I held his hand and stayed up with him the last hours of his death. His imprint will always be in my memory.

Richard

His name is Richard. He is mean and ugly. Apparently he has always been very independent. He suffered a stroke. He is a big man and reminds me of a hunchback. He is angry at his wife all the time for having placed him in the home, but she simply couldn't take his meanness anymore. At first he wanted to prove he could still care for himself, but the problem was he couldn't do anything with his hands. He fought everyone off and tried to take a stab at me with his fork. One day he choked on a piece of meat and I ran to assist him and was able to dislodge the obstructing piece from his throat. Later he thanked me and told me I had saved his life. His attitude has changed and I have earned his trust. Later he became more involved, cooperative, and pleasant.

Pauline

She is always one who is demanding—and sometimes rude. Taking care of her is a chore every night. I came to work one day and stopped by the living room as there was a movie on— the movie was a war movie and while I was not interested, Pauline was there taking it all in. After the movie, Pauline was taken to her room where I found her on my 3:00 p.m. rounds. She was sitting in the corner, very quiet and staring into space. I asked her how she was and she looked at me and burst into tears. She told me she should never have gone, because it brought back memories of the son she had lost in the war. I felt so much compassion for her that I took her in my arms and shared her sorrow. That's when I knew that she had a soft heart—we both cried and she became my friend because she shared her secret with me.

Soap operas on television don't even come close to capturing the intensity of the moments, the sharing of pain, and the delight of new relationships and loss of others which are part of the nursing home drama. Visitors, uncomfortable with their images and feelings, sometimes fail to witness these touching and moving exchanges between aides and residents. Brief 15 to 30 minute visits in a nursing home will not reveal the daily drama in all its glory. Visitors must come regularly and often to discover the humanness that gets exchanged.

One day David took a break from a week-long class he was conducting in a Kansas nursing home. He sat down next to Ethel, an aide of 20 years on the skilled care wing. Both were sipping sodas when David asked, "Ethel, how do you do it?"

"Do what?" she responded.

"How do you live and work on this floor, with the most difficult patients, some who are uncommunicative, and most who don't remember your name, and stay sane?" David replied.

"What makes you think it is difficult?"

"Well," he said, "I think it would be difficult to come to work day in and day out and try to relate to what appears to be some hopeless cases. I think I would get discouraged and depressed."

"Actually, it is quite easy loving these people," she said with conviction. "I just look past the wrinkles and see the soul."

Nursing assistants who work daily with persons who are physically less than what they used to be, encounter more than anyone else the spirit or the life of being. The resident lies naked before the aide. All the secrets and masks which once served as protection against societal and other evaluations are exposed and drawn aside. The love and affection which gets exchanged then is based on meanings and understandings not often found in the "outside" world, but which are commonplace in the world of the nursing home. Older people in the home are loved for their humanness and their vulnerability, not for their external appearances. It is fascinating that entry-level, less skilled workers are more likely to experience this than other, more educated, supervisory personnel. It may be that "lower-level" workers, having also experienced oppression and a sense of abandonment, have a greater affinity with the persons for whom they care than those who, in life, have been more fortunate.

An aide shared this moment with David:

> I was working with Lorine one day, a victim of Alzheimer's Disease. She was crying and very unwilling to let me take care of her. I put my arms around her and told her I loved her, and she said she loved me too. She calmed down and let me give her the care she needed. I realized she needs to be told she is loved. We all need to be loved. I find it easy to tell her, "I love you," because I do. And she loves me back, even if she doesn't know it.

Chapter Six

Administrators, Supervisors, and the Underground

While the caregivers are a special group, the nursing home environment cannot function without upper staff — those holding the top positions in the hierarchy. Administrators and supervisors deserve special mention. Their world is unique for they have their own set of problems and frustrations.

Any home, whether a proprietary or a not-for-profit facility, must fill beds in order to stay in business. Balancing resources and the cost of care is the constant struggle of the administrator. If a sufficient number of beds is not filled, that is, if "census" is down, tension goes up throughout the facility. This seems to be a universal law in nursing homes. Worse, the tension has a "trickle down" effect as it first affects supervisors who may have to begin the process of selecting which staff to "let go." This in turn affects staff at all levels who may be the ones selected. The formula for success is to keep all the beds filled so there will be plenty of resources to provide the finest care. Lose patients, and cost will exceed resources and subsequently jeopardize quality of care. It is a delicate balancing act which only those close to the top fully appreciate and understand.

Supervisory personnel have the dual and often untenable role of grasping and accepting the realities of census and financial matters, yet with limited resources they are expected to maintain the highest professional standards and quality care in their areas. Their education and training create the assumption that the necessary resources will be provided, but this is rarely the case in a nursing home.

The "underground" is the name we have given to an unacknowledged but vital force within nursing homes. In a small home, it may include administrative and supervisory personnel, but more often, it is a hidden factor composed of a mixture of middle-level and lower-level employees who do both the work they are hired to do and their own "secret service."

ADMINISTRATORS

The administrator, dreading the worst, opens the note which has been quietly handed to her during the seminar.

> Mrs. Becker—
> I'm sorry to bother you, but the air conditioner has broken down again. Everyone is hot and tempers are beginning to get unbearable. I think you had better get back to town quick!
>
> Gail

Mary Becker sat still for several minutes pondering her next move. For months now she has been looking forward to the California trip, and the educational seminar sponsored by the American College of Health Care Administrators is living up to all of her expectations. She slowly turns in her chair and says to no one in particular, "Damn. I've got to leave. The health inspectors are due any time and they will never understand this one."

She slowly pushes away from the table, turns over her licensure credit sign-in sheet, and carefully slips out the door trying not to disturb the session.

"Why me? Why now?" Mrs. Becker whines silently as she walks to the fancy pay phone hanging on the wall. "Why did I ever get into this business in the first place?" she asks for the hundredth time.

"Hello Gail, this is Mary. Give me the details." Mary sounds more like a mother than an administrator of a 200-bed nursing care facility. But then, Gail, her new assistant administrator-in-training, sometimes seemed more like her child than her fellow professional. There had been an element of risk in going off and leaving Gail in charge—not a risk if events moved in everyday fashion, but only if the dreaded major happening occurred. And now it had.

"I think the motor burned out. Larry heard a small explosion and found evidence of what must have been a brief fire. At any rate, the wires are charred, we have called 'Inferno Controllers,' and several of our faithful volunteers are rounding up some fans." Clearly exhausted, Gail waits for her boss to provide the next direction.

"The inspectors are due anytime, you know." Mrs. Becker now sounds like the administrator. Gail knows she is beginning to marshall her managerial forces. "I'll be there by 9 o'clock tonight. Put Larry in charge of the air conditioner, and you take charge of all the staff, not just nursing personnel. If we're lucky, the inspectors won't notice a thing."

Mary clicks the phone and quickly places a call to the airport. The emergency plan is set in motion.

"It's the regulations that get to you," she tries to explain to her seat companion on the flight home. "We have to make good on over 500 items or risk losing our license. If we lose our license, we lose our residents. And if we lose our residents, we go out of business. And if we go out of business, we have to put the residents on the street. Thus my first priority is to stay OPEN. Anything that threatens that means going home to fight the good fight. That's why I must return."

"Why can't you delegate your responsibilities to others at the home?" the companion inquires.

"I have good staff. And often I do count on them to keep things running smoothly. But the buck stops here. If deficiencies are not met, it is my fault. If residents leave, it is my fault. If staff doesn't show up for work, it is my fault. If the food tastes lousy, it is my fault. If the air conditioner doesn't work, it is my fault." Mary stops her rhythmic flow for she realizes that it can go on forever.

"I don't think I would want your job!" the fellow passenger exclaims as she turns to look at the patchwork fields below.

Mary retreats too. Her mind slowly sinks into a stream of consciousness filled with air conditioners, nursing pools, family complainers, lawyers, insurance agents, and inspectors. For nearly an hour she can think of nothing but problems. "Why do I do this?" she wonders. "I am an administrator because I care about people," she reminds herself. "I do care about people . . . Oh how I miss Mrs. Abernathy . . . I wonder if she is still recovering from her fall

. . . And Mr. Bell. I wonder if his family took him for a ride yesterday. They said they would . . . but of course they have said that before."

Mary's mind is still racing. The threat of being given a deficiency by the inspectors for improper temperature control and ventilation has all but devastated what was otherwise a peaceful respite from the everyday trials and tribulations of running a nursing home. What makes nursing home management such an unpredictable occupation is the fact that every day is a new day. A smart administrator will include in his or her schedule time for the unexpected. A lot of time.

"Oh, my gosh," Mary almost blurts her thought into the cabin, "Those people must be burning up!" Mary can't believe it. This is the first time that the residents have crossed her mind. She is so preoccupied with regulations, standards, and survival, she almost forgets about the people as she cares about most. "The fans will never do it. It's nearly 100 degrees outside and, as usual, yesterday's rain will bring the humidity to unbearable levels." She grips the armrest feeling powerless to relieve the suffering of her people.

"LADIES AND GENTLEMEN, WE ARE BEGINNING OUR DESCENT INTO KANSAS CITY, PLEASE FASTEN YOUR SEAT BELTS AND BRING ALL TRAY TABLES AND CHAIRS INTO THEIR UPRIGHT POSITION. WE WILL BE AT THE GATE IN APPROXIMATELY SEVEN MINUTES." Mrs. Becker dutifully secures her area and person, but quickly returns to the flow of her previous thoughts.

"Yes, I care. But I never have a chance to spend much time with my people. I'm always into things, things, things, not people. Air conditioners, food trays, wheelchairs, and exit signs, not people. Regs, rules, and site visits, not people. Beds and bedpans, not people. Oh, how I miss my people," she laments. "Why, I see people on the floors who know me, but I don't have the faintest idea who they are . . . what has happened?"

"How big is your nursing home?" the passenger interrupts as the plane makes its final approach.

"We have 200 beds and 192 of them filled," Mary answers with a sense of pride. After all, the home had only 62% occupancy when she took over less than two years ago.

"That's quite a few souls to take care of, isn't it?" the lady responds as she answers her own question.

"It sure is," replies Mary, "but I only had 32 persons to take care of in my first job."

Mary hears her own statement as if it is broadcast over the loudspeaker. "That's it," she thinks. "When I had the small home, the problems were the same, but the job was more fun. And there was more time for people. It was very different from what I have now. Maybe nursing homes should reach a certain optimal size and then be forced to start a new one once the limit has been reached. The Israelis learned that years ago with their Kibbutzim . . . If we could only afford to do it," Mary sighs in despair.

"WELCOME TO KANSAS CITY. THE TEMPERATURE IS A WARM 95 DEGREES AT 7:30 P.M., CENTRAL DAY-LIGHT TIME. IF YOU ARE LEAVING US HERE, WE WISH YOU A WONDERFUL STAY IN THIS UP-TO-DATE, ALL-AMERICAN CITY."

"Up-to-date is right. My nursing home is up-to-date, but the general public still has such a negative attitude toward what we try to do," Mary says to her companion.

"I honestly don't know how you can work there," replies the lady.

"Case closed," Mary tries to say cheerfully.

Mary Becker was particularly disappointed that she had to leave the professional seminar in California. What the American public fails to realize is the extent to which the long-term health care field goes to enhance the professional growth of its leaders. Three national groups continue to make their imprint on the profession: the American Health Care Association, the American Association of Homes for the Aged, and the American College of Health Care Administrators. Each of these groups, and countless community colleges, four-year colleges, and universities hold professional seminars for administrators, nurses, activity directors, and even occasional events for entry-level personnel. All administrators are required to pass state licensure requirements and to renew this certification every two years by attending continuing education events approved for licensure credit. Currently, there are no such requirements for administrators of acute care hospitals in America.

What Mary Becker missed most was not necessarily the credit she would have to make up elsewhere, but rather the quality of the program being offered in California. In such a rapidly growing and changing field, it is critical to stay informed and on top of your profession. Many administrators like Mary often accumulate far more hours than required for licensure credit. There is much to know and so little time to learn it.

Because the world of the nursing home is so different from the world of the hospital and other health care related institutions, it requires special training. Patients in a nursing home are not expected to be passive and confined, but rather active and unrestrained. The administrative model of organization in a hospital often stops with department heads and budgets, but in the nursing home it extends to personalities and families. Children "under age 14" are not only permitted, they are encouraged and enjoyed by all in the nursing home. And finally, in the nursing home it is an interdisciplinary team, rather than the physician, who determines and executes care plans.

Often it is difficult for an individual to cross over from hospital-based experience and training into the world of the nursing home. The transition is not an easy one. All the expectations, of both staff and patient, change. The so-called "medical model" simply does not fit the needs of residents. This is most dramatically experienced when a newly hired Director of Nurses, trained only in a hospital, enters a nursing home for the first time. All kinds of reverberations can occur. No wonder nurses' aides (the least trained employees) sometimes feel they know more about caring for the patients than their supervisors. They have learned, through experience, that the "medical model" is inadequate in a nursing home. A more holistic approach to caring is required instead. This means that those who work in this environment must know more, and be prepared for more, than those who work in the prestigious hospital across town. It takes a special personality.

Perhaps the administrator needs to be a giant of a person. He or she must have a thorough knowledge of public policy in long-term care (particularly knowledge about Medicare, Medicaid, and other reimbursement plans), an understanding of 468 diagnostic related groups of health conditions (a Dangerous Roulette Game that the

Health Care Financing Administration currently advocates), and a knowledge of all guaranteed "patient rights." He or she must be a great communicator who relates well with other administrators, staff, families, and residents themselves, a business manager, a leader who initiates action rather than one who passively responds to one crisis after another, an individual who understands and can appropriate an interdisciplinary model of care. He or she must have a sense of humor and be visible in his or her own nursing home as well as in the community. In short, it is not an easy job. In fact, if one considers it a job, as opposed to a career, he or she will not last long. This is clearly a 24 hour per day commitment. Anything short of this will not get the job done.

SUPERVISORS

RNs

We finish our lunch and our mutual updating, and settle back for a long talk over our iced tea. The restaurant is not crowded, there is no pressure to leave. Now we can discuss our shared past as head floor nurses at Raven Hill Nursing and Health Care Center with all the honesty and insight that time and distance have given us.

"Those first few months at the nursing home were some of the hardest of my nursing career, Marian. Being a hospital RN hadn't prepared me for long-term care realities. In the hospital, I sent people home well or improved for the most part. Death wasn't really such a constant factor. Those first months at Raven I lost five people on my floor! And neither my professional training nor my faith seemed to help me deal with it."

Marian nods her understanding. "It became worse," she says, "with the DRGs. On my skilled care floor, we would get sick, old people who had been dismissed from the hospital because their DRG time had run out. Sometimes we'd have to send them back to the hospital the next day—or worse, they'd die within 24 hours. That just traumatized me, professionally and personally. No amount of rationalizing about it helped. I am a nurse and I'm supposed to make people better. It took me a long time to learn to take satisfaction from the fact that I could see they were made comfortable and treated compassionately.''

We are each wound up in our own "house of horrors" now. I speak again.

"The very worst for me—the thing that had me calling for the chaplain, was being able to look at some of my patients and know they would be dead, say of another stroke, within a few months, and that there was nothing medically we could do about it. Having that kind of knowledge hurt like hell and threw me off balance, as you say, both professionally and personally. I did eventually make an adjustment of sorts, but sometimes I wanted to curse my medical competence.''

Marian laughs dryly. "You've hit it, Georgia, the 'RNs' Curse'— medical competence! Isn't that what often makes our days a battlefield with our old nemesis, the physician? We can know as much medically as they do, and certainly we know the patients better because we're with them, observing them, daily, hourly, but we're rarely accepted as equals. We both remember residents we lost because we couldn't get a doctor to take some action or to stop some action. You, at least, were usually honest and straightforward with them.''

"It didn't help much," I respond. "The patient was just as sick or as dead as if I'd said nothing."

We drink our teas, each absorbed in memories of incidents that still haunt us. Marian speaks again.

"I don't think I ever tried harder than I did with the aides on my floor at Raven, but essentially, I failed. Oh, I got rid of a few bad apples, and some of the care improved, but I never did win their trust and wholehearted cooperation. I believe so in the importance of their role, and I brought them into decision-making as much as I could, but they were never really 'with me'." Marian smiles wryly. "Mostly, I remember incidents like the one with Doris Blake during that bad outbreak of staph infection. When I ordered the aides to put on protective paper gowns, gloves, and shoe covers—as much for their own protection as the patients', I overheard Doris mutter, 'Why do we have a staph problem anyway if she's (meaning me) so smart and educated?'''

I smile. "Well, that's part of it, of course. When there are differing levels of education, the ones who have more are sometimes resented—particularly if they're in the 'boss' role as we are. I think aides often view us as smart, but lacking common sense as they see it. I didn't have as much trouble as you did because I come basically from the same background as they do. I know what their lives are like and what pressures they're under, but I always took the stand that once inside the nursing home and on my floor, the standards and practices I set were to be followed. I meant business and they knew it. I was hard on them, but fair, and they knew I wasn't above helping out no matter what the job. In the end, of course, it was because of the aides that I resigned. Whatever decisions the administration made, it seemed to me the aides ended up bearing the brunt of it and none of my efforts on their behalf did any good."

The waitress, despairing of our departure, refills our glasses once again.

"Ah, Administration," Marian sighs. "There's the real rub. I recall the beautiful spiel I was given about my job and how creative and independent they wanted me to be on my floor. And I was, too! My floor really became 'home' to those residents. They were being active in ways they hadn't been since coming to the home. Then the administrator calls me in and says, 'We're cutting positions for budget reasons; yours is one, so we're letting you go. You can resign if that's helpful.' Not a word about any of my accomplishments, no sense of valuing what I'd tried to do!"

I reach over and squeeze Marian's hand. "And you had done a special thing, Marian. We 'floor people' knew it, but the 'office folks' rarely know much of value, anyway. What finally got to me was the way the money was allocated. Everything was painted and made beautiful on the outside—new furniture, refurbished dining area—all impressive to potential residents and families. But at the same time, I lacked supplies and sufficient aides to properly care for people. And I just saw no way out of those conflicting value systems."

Across the table, Marian smiles. "This is doing me a world of good, Georgia. I've needed to get this out of my system ever since I left Raven. And I've got another group that drives me up the wall—families. Take Mr. Whelan. We'd worked with him for a month getting his diabetes under control, hoping to save him from a future loss of a foot or worse. He'd really adjusted to his new diet, was making friends and going to activities. Then his wife started read-dicting him by smuggling in cookies. The neurotic pattern they'd worked out in their marriage was about broken and I guess she felt, in her sick way, that she was losing him. The social worker and I did our best, but in the end Mrs. Whelan won. She convinced him we were the 'meanies' and he turned back into a miserable, dissatis-fied grouch."

I chuckle now with hindsight, recalling the many tirades of which I had been the target. "I think I averaged about two abusive calls a week from families. I really wanted families to come to me with problems and complaints. I always told them so during our initial interview and meant it. For some that was all that was needed. They knew the home's limitations and my own, and within that frame-work, we worked things out. But, the demanding ones, the guilty ones! Even though I understood them, the abuse was hard to take. I didn't want my staff to bear the brunt of it; the buck stopped with me as head nurse. As with your Mr. Whelan, the really sad part was when a physician and the family would take someone out of the home where they were loved and would have been comfortable, and put them in the hospital just to die."

The noon crowd has long gone from the restaurant. We glance guiltily at our resigned waitress, but are determined to toast our last group—the residents.

"I was absolutely crazy about most of them," I say. "Many of them were more relaxed and frank when dealing with the head nurse, so I often saw the best side of them. They could be rather high handed with the aides at times. Some, of course, saw me as their personal servant. Remember Mrs. Allison, who used to have me paged over the loud speaker when she wanted fresh water?"

Marian laughs. "I remember. And I had some wonderful charac-ters and some real sweethearts on my floor. But, I never got to know many residents as well as the other staff did. I usually knew medical histories better than personal ones, which makes me feel guilty."

"Well, I'm feeling guilty about the waitress," I respond. "Let's go and leave her a guilt-sized tip!"

LPNs

"I became an aide because I didn't have much choice. But I found I loved nursing, and I chose to become an LPN. I'm proud to be one.

"Being an LPN is a little like being the filling in a sandwich with bread pressing down on the top and up from the bottom. We LPNs are in the middle, and that's not easy.

"I've respected a lot of RNs and been friends with one, but mostly I think of myself as working 'under' them. For a good part of the time they're not around; they're in their office or in some meeting. And that means I'm in charge without really being in charge. I mean — I must see that everything is done, supervising the aides, calling the doctors about patient problems or to get orders, but no one really sees me as the boss. Some of the doctors are o.k. — they ask questions and treat you as if you had some sense. But others seem annoyed that a lowly LPN is calling to make a request and they let you know it. I have to be very, very careful to be accurate about the information I give and the information I receive. I'm the 'go-between.' If the RN doesn't include some needed fact, the doctor blames me. And if the doctor doesn't give good instructions, it looks like I wasn't listening well. On really busy days, I'm exhausted from the tension of being sure I get everything right.

"The same is true with the paper work and keeping the charts up. This is our job and it has to be thorough and accurate or mistakes could get residents or staff in real trouble.

"Having been an aide myself, I knew the kind of trouble to expect there. Some aides look down on any other aide who has ambition and becomes an LPN. They think she's gone 'high hat,' and there's no convincing them otherwise. Some of them think you ought to do your old job of being an aide *and* your new one as LPN. Well, if I'd wanted to be an aide, I would have stayed an aide! But, it's not their fault that there aren't enough of them to do a really good job. Some days are really bad for them. I try to help out, but I've got my own job to do. When I have to train aides, I sometimes feel their resentment or I get disgusted with those that don't really care to learn. It's just a paycheck to some of them.

"I'm also responsible for medicines and treatments if that's my assignment. Again, I have to concentrate and be very accurate. Some people see that concentration as unfriendliness. You can't win.

"I love the residents and wish I had more time with them. On one job I did have more time and I would organize sing-a-longs or just visit. That's the way it ought to be.

"Don't ask me about administration. I hardly recognize those people when I see them. If they'd get off what they sit on and spend some real time on the floor, we'd all be better off."

THE ACTIVITY DIRECTOR

Marge stood reading the carefully typed note signed with the familiar bold pen of the administrator. As the knot tightened in her stomach, she observed how the apparent simplicity of the message seemed undone by the power and impatience of the signature scrawled at the bottom of the page.

"Marge," it read, "Channel 7 wants to interview four or five residents about their childhood experiences of Christmas. I know you will select people who will do us proud. Please see that they are appropriately dressed and ready in the lobby by eleven tomorrow morning. Thanks, as always, (signed) Evelyn." Crushing the note in her hand, Marge headed for the sanctuary of her office on the lower level of Deacon Manor.

Everything, she thought — and knew she was being accurate as well as bitter — falls into the Activity Director's lap. Whenever they didn't know what to do with something or no one else had time for it, they passed it on to her. I'm the dumping ground, she repeated to herself; it had become her inner theme song.

This particular assignment, however, was more painful than usual, robbing her of her own plans for the residents this afternoon. She had carefully set aside several hours when she could take her guitar and give herself fully to visiting the bedridden on the skilled care wing. The unmet needs of these people for human contact and live entertainment haunted her. Although a few of them might respond to the bedside activities she had learned at a recent workshop, she suspected most would prefer the gift of a personal exchange. She had planned to sit and visit, and then ask for a song request which she would do specially for the resident or perhaps get the resident to join with her in the singing. Marge had fantasized the scene with pleasure: music would surely draw an aide into the room and they would all share in the song and the fellowship. It would be an afternoon of building those personal bonds and ties which she believed to be the essence of her job and the fulfillment of her purpose to provide activity and enrichment to the lives of the residents at Deacon.

Her afternoon's plans were shot, of course. She could think of two "dependables" — residents who were articulate and enjoyed public appearances. She could enlist them quickly, she hoped. But, Marge could sense the problems that lay ahead as she ticked possible choices off on her fingers.

Mr. Hazlett was chancy. He could be delightful and fit for TV consumption on his good days, but she couldn't count on tomorrow being a good day. On his "off" days, he rambled on and on about nocturnal visits from his long dead mother. It was hard to know if Mr. Hazlett found these visitations a comfort or a curse. She herself found it all rather touching, but it was no more what Channel 7 and Evelyn were seeking than the Ghost of Christmas Past had been in Scrooge's nighttime plans.

Mrs. Bradley would be wonderful, but "froze" in any kind of formal situation. Marge groaned at the recollection of the time Mrs. Bradley had been elected Deacon's Mother of the Year. At the Mother's Day Tea, Marge had been forced to cajole Mrs. B. into telling about her experiences of motherhood and about her children. It was hard to know which of them had been more humiliated as they stood at the head of the table with Mrs. Bradley stammering and mumbling in miserable embarrassment. Certainly no one had been entertained.

For her other selections, Marge knew she must count on help from the nurses. If they were enthused about one of their people being on TV, they would be wonderfully helpful in the selection and preparation of the resident. Still, Marge knew the better part of the afternoon must now be given over to persuasion and perhaps tracking down a suitable outfit for a TV appearance.

Marge's eye was caught by Monday's note which she had impaled with distaste on the spindle. It was Administration's suggested list of name changes for her job. She glanced at them: Director of Community Living, Director of Social and Religious Services, Director of Community Relations. Mouthfuls all and impressive. Director of Social and Religious Services was certainly the most accurate. Seeing to the religious needs of residents by organizing services and calling pastors and churches for classes and program commitments was a feature of her role about which she felt inadequate. What she needed to do, she thought, was to push hard for at least a part-time chaplain who would take on some of the religious load.

Taking her sandwich and apple from the brown paper bag, Marge settled back to mull over what she wanted to change about her job. For certain, she would do away with or greatly modify some of the traditional festivities. Neither the families nor the residents enjoyed them much—except for the proffered food. Even the fashion show last year, which appeared to be a great success, was debatable. There were inevitably hurt feelings because staff selected the residents who were to "walk the runway." Some residents and families, Marge felt, had been somewhat manipulated in order to see that a good-looking outfit would be worn by the "model." The residents had looked marvelous—dressed up and made up—and the audience had been delighted with the spectacle, but it *had* been a spectacle.

Marge thought of the three events that had been thoroughly satisfying and successful, and realized that they had all been grassroots initiated and spontaneous. There had been the day on the Second Floor when the nurses and residents had gathered in the dining area for a distribution of donated clothes. It had had all the fun and excitement of a shopping spree without the crowds or the cost.

And there had been the party given on a Friday afternoon by the First Floor staff just because they wanted to do something fun with the people they cared for. It had been a real party—you could feel it.

Marge recalled the pleasure of a Christmas morning on the

Fourth Floor when the nurses had brought in the breakfast makings and cooked right there in the dining room. With residents milling about in their bathrobes and the enticing smells, it had been like a Christmas morning at home.

That's it, Marge thought. I'll ask that my title be changed to Director of Human Services, and I'll spend my time stimulating and encouraging grassroots activities. She wadded-up her brown paper bag and tossed it at the wastepaper basket. It struck the side and fell to the floor. Her request, she thought, would go into the wastebasket and stay there.

Good thinking, Marge, but not realistic, she sighed to herself. She took out the official book in which she was required to keep a record of each resident and how often they attended activities. The state inspector poured over this. She saw that Charlie Herndon's page was blank as usual. The state wouldn't accept the fact that Charlie had been a loner all of his life and totally natural and content in his own company.

Allowing people to be human was the hardest activity of all, Marge thought as she headed to locate five new TV stars.

SOCIAL WORKERS, CHAPLAINS, AND OTHERS

There are, of course, other actors in this drama. While the great majority of nursing homes do not have full-time social workers, chaplains, dentists, occupational therapists, music specialists, and others, many do have persons who work on a part-time basis, travel between facilities, or volunteer to provide these kinds of services.

Social workers are particularly skilled in getting the story and saying "Hello in there" to residents who need to feel valued. Unfortunately, much of their time is spent with admissions, early adjustment problems, paperwork, recertification decisions, and with serious conflicts which may emerge between families, staff, and residents. One-on-one private time with those who live and work in the home is often limited.

Full-time chaplains are currently a rarity in the long-term health care field. In fact, the spiritual dimension of self is perhaps the most neglected and least nourished facet of the wonderfully frail older persons who live in nursing homes. Residents who can leave to attend the community worship service of their choice are lucky. Others must usually make due with an ecumenical series of rotating ministers who volunteer their services over the course of the year. There may be a bible study class (or its equivalent) from time to time. But it is certain that a good portion of residents will never again experience the fellowship of a church community. Spirituality remains an individual matter, and while God often pulls these residents through, the miracles go unnoticed and are rarely shared. While we anticipate that every nursing home in America will someday have a chaplain, it cannot happen soon enough.

Occupational therapists will appear with greater frequency as the vertical integration of services (home health care, adult day care, etc.) offered by hospitals, and as subacute (rehabilitative) care in nursing homes, continues. These persons add a special dimension to long-term care. When residents can spend time using old and developing new skills in creating and producing, everyone benefits. The resident often experiences a higher degree of self-esteem, staff becomes attentive and responsive to the work of the resident, and family members and others begin to realize that there are things to do in a nursing home. Perhaps best of all, activities planned and directed by an occupational therapist give the resident something to look forward to, indeed, something to wake up for.

Dentists for teeth, podiatrists for feet, and barbers and cosmetologists for hair, make their appearances too. These services often get offered in any number and variety of ways; it is unfortunate, however, when they are not offered. Losing dentures, or imagining that they have been stolen, can be very frustrating. Moreover, a large proportion of older persons need dental work whether they are in a nursing home or not. Although a feeling of personal attractiveness may be in jeopardy for the resident, it is often families and nutritionists who react negatively as older persons resist the discomfort of dentures that cannot be redone often enough to keep pace with changes in the mouth cavity. Teeth should not go untended.

Nonambulatory persons often have difficulty caring for the feet which once carried them to the far reaches of their personal and professional worlds. Residents in nursing homes are quite aware that outsiders often respond negatively to ugly toenails and feet.

And for those who still walk, keeping the feet fit may be the most important health care treatment in the smorgasbord of services offered. Ingrown toenails, poor circulation, and infection can be the forerunners of more serious medical problems.

As for their hair, our obvious preoccupation with "how it looks" should give some clue as to how important it remains for those who are now living in nursing homes. For women in our culture, attractive hair is essential to a good presentation of self. Wrinkles and weight may not be within a woman's control, but hair can remain her crowning glory. Beauty and barber shops (or the nursing home facsimiles thereof) provide grooming opportunities, but very often the same room is used for both men and women. This can, of course, be very demeaning to men who remember and relate to the barber shop as if it were a sacred place of worship. For many men, the barber shop was a place you could go to talk about sex, baseball, politics, and religion . . . in that order! The haircut, if you got one, was only secondary. Fellowship was primary.

There are other services offered to nursing home residents, but what seems missing in almost every case is the social activity and contagion which often surrounds such "treatments" when they are offered in the outside world. Even mealtime, which was once a psychosocial drama, can become simply a nutritional event. Volunteers are desperately needed in nursing homes to assist and help in providing these and other services. And what the volunteer needs to know is that important as it is that the teeth get cleaned, the toenails get cut, the hair gets combed, the pottery gets fired, and the soul gets blessed, it is equally important that someone be there to share with residents these everyday activities of being human.

THE UNDERGROUND

David has observed it; Sally has participated in it. The nursing home underground is a genuine phenomenon. It takes a number of forms. It can simply be individuals who, unofficially and unauthorized, become real forces in the lives of residents. It can also be a casual come-and-go coalition of unrelated staff members who take power which no one else wants, and use it. The common denominator here is humanness — people working directly with and for other people. Administrators and supervisors are often unaware of this force until its strength and influence confront them through some incident.

Housekeeping was a major force in the underground in Sally's nursing home. After the first resident death of her chaplaincy, Sally brought the family to her "desk and chair" office for privacy in their grief and a quiet place to make decisions and phone calls. The next day, the head housekeeper appeared at Sally's door and said, "If you're going to be using this office for people like that, it's got to be better than it is now. I've located a couch, some chairs, tables, and lamps. Can I send them up this afternoon?" All unasked for, all unauthorized—all underground.

A workshop with housekeeping employees turned out to be one of the most revealing and inspiring of Sally's chaplaincy. This group included room and bathroom cleaners (from dignified great-grandmothers to pregnant young women) and floor moppers (mostly young men). They came reluctantly because it cut into their break time. Some came skeptically ("What's she going to do?") and others, suspiciously ("Is she going to talk religion?"). But when the key question was asked—"Tell me, who are your favorite residents?"—another layer of the rich underground life of the nursing home was uncovered.

One young man had his own special group whom he saw daily. These were mostly men termed "difficult" by the staff. They were not "difficult" for the young floor cleaner—they were delightful and cherished friends. One difficult resident who was so reluctant a verbal communicator that most of the staff dealt with him only by gesture, talked freely and happily during his daily visits with the floor cleaner. This same young employee confessed somewhat shyly that each day he bought and delivered a Coke to a lady resident who waited eagerly for his arrival.

One of the most dignified of the women housekeepers remained silent and solemn until the hour was almost ended. Then she blurted out, "Oh, I know nobody likes her! But, Thelma is my favorite." Her look defied any of us to say a critical word. "We have long, very private conversations while I clean her room. People say she weeps over nothing. But, I understand her. Sometimes weeping is just weeping.'' In the presence of such understanding and compassion, everyone was respectfully silent.

The housekeeping employees' supervisor had been seated inconspicuously in the room listening. When her people had returned to work, she confessed to Sally that while she had been aware that her staff had favorites, she had no idea of the depth of their involvement.

In the nursing home where Sally worked, a woman in the business office was a key member of the underground. For years she had helped residents with their business and personal affairs. Many residents considered her their best friend. Most visited her daily. Money was lent. Cigarettes and sweaters were bought. Bills were explained. Phone calls were made to straighten out problems. A skeptical resident finally accepted the fact that her old home was uninhabitable only after her friend in the business office visited it and told her so. Staff came to the woman in the business office for information and assistance with residents. Families beat a path to her desk to have complicated business affairs reduced to intelligibility.

Mostly unaware and all unbelieving, Administration, during a major shifting of offices, placed this underground heroine's office in a remote and inaccessible corner of the nursing home. All hell broke loose. It was as though a death had occurred. The pattern of the real life of the nursing home had been violated and Administration had no choice but to return this key person to the major traffic area so that life could be resumed.

A death in the nursing home can also be disruptive. A resident's only child refused to claim her mother's body. The daughter washed her hands of any responsibility. So, the aforementioned woman in the business office, the telephone operator/receptionist (another key member of this nursing home underground), and Sally formed a triumvirate to see that the deceased resident was properly and lovingly buried. The woman in the business office located an undertaker willing to do an inexpensive but dignified burial. A cemetery plot was similarly found. The receptionist spread the message of needed contributions. Staff, residents, and their families (including the five-year-old great-grandson of the deceased resident's roommate) gave happily and generously to the fund. Finally, Sally performed the graveside funeral service on a morning when a light snow had wrapped the cemetery in white serenity. The underground had done its work.

PART III: TRANSFORMATION

Chapter Seven

Celebration

In Chapter One we brought you through the doors into the world of the nursing home. In Chapters Two and Three we faced head-on some of the frustrations and anxieties this experience can be for many people. Part II of the book explored the personal and professional worlds of nursing assistants, supervisory personnel, administrators, and those we chose to call the "underground." The intent has been to bring the reader through the initial horror of the nursing home and into its humanness. While special moments have been illustrated from time to time, we now wish to bring to the surface this humanness which struggles to be seen and experienced. The many players in this drama have their special problems with which to deal, but it is undeniable that the human spirit is present in nursing homes. This chapter celebrates the humanness in these settings.

ANNE REVISITED

Even now, six months after Dad's death and two years after making the decision to place him in a nursing home, I am uncertain of his real feelings about that initial move. On his "good days," as I bustled about his house, discussing with him what he wanted to take with him, he seemed reconciled and accepting of the idea that it was "the only thing to do." On those days, I felt like Annie again—

Annie, his beloved child and companion, whom he trusted implicitly and whom he believed had made the right decision for him. On other days when age and poor health seemed to place Dad in a world I could not enter, I would catch him looking at me as though I were indeed Anne, his Executioner. My heart would grow cold in me, and with guilt and grief. I would again rush at him with logic and reason, hoping to win back my Annie status. But this man was both my father and a stranger—an ambivalence that neither love nor reason seemed to resolve.

The first two months of Dad's nursing home residency were traumatic for me. My bewilderment at who my father had become was nothing compared to the total confusion about who I now was. When Dad had been at home, I had been "it"—his caretaker, his protector, his decision-maker, his confidante, his companion. I had not sought these roles, but they had become so ingrained in me that in spite of the fact that I had put Dad in a nursing home so that others could give him better care, I continued to act as caregiver. Nurses reassured me and my family pointed out the absurdity of my behavior, but in spite of the burdens, the ego satisfaction of Dad's dependence on me had become my "meat and potatoes." It took an incident to shock me into awareness.

I had come early, bearing tidbits of news to entertain Dad and homemade cookies to feed him. Dad's roommate was gone and the curtain between their beds was pulled out, hiding Dad and the aide from my sight. I stood and listened.

Aide: "I swear, Mr. Bronson, you've got the toughest beard I *ever* tried to shave! Don't you know that?"

Dad: "Mae, I've never shaved anyone else but myself, so how would I know? You're the expert here."

Mae: "That's what I'm telling you: I'm the expert here, and I say you've got the toughest beard I ever shaved and you better hold still if you don't want to look like you'd run into a thorn bush!" They laughed happily.

Dad: "O.K., Mae, I'll hold still. In fact, if you do a good job, I'll share the cookies from the birthday party which I stashed away last night."

Mae: "Now, Mr. B., your memory's playing tricks on you

again. There wasn't a birthday party last night — so no cookies to stash. But, I'll tell you what. When we finish here, I have my break. I'll get a package of those chocolate chip cookies we both like from the machine and bring you some when I come back."

Dad: "Fair enough, Mae. But, remember, I want a real cookie and not just some crumbs from yours!" They laughed again.

I experienced a wave of jealousy so intense it took my breath away. I turned and left, hurrying from the building as fast as I could. Bitter tears of grief and loss exploded as I reached the privacy of my car. The reality of what had been happening during the last three months in the nursing home washed over me, rinsing away my self-imposed blinders and restoring my sight. In the hours of thought and reflection that followed, this is what I "saw."

Dad was better; not well, not cured, but better in the nursing home environment than he had been at home with me looking after him. He was protected from many of the things that had been hurtful like ordering and reordering his groceries. In spite of my seeming acceptance of his memory problems, he had sensed underneath my words, the disappointment, fear, and yes, anger. In the nursing home his memory loss was accepted as genuinely O.K. — that is, as nothing to be uptight about, but unthreatening and often humorous. It would be many months before I, as daughter, could even approximate such an attitude. Which led me to another insight.

Notwithstanding the family's love and devotion, Dad needed new friends. Yes, at 78, Dad needed new friends. Not his children, in-laws, and grandchildren who remembered him as he was in his prime, and who mourned the loss of what he had been. Not his Annie, who hated and feared the changes in him, and at times even tried to force him to be what he no longer was. Mae and the other people in the nursing home made friends with a man who was charming, humorous, usually cooperative, but sometimes quarrelsome and depressed. They all liked him and a few loved him. They were unburdened by the loss of the wise and supportive father, the sharp-minded and companionable father-in-law, the loving and interested grandfather. And he, in turn, was not burdened with false expectations. He could be the best of what he was with them. It took many more months before I could relax and accept Dad sufficiently to enjoy not baking cookies for him, but sharing the machine-bought chocolate chips with him on a day when he could not recall his granddaughter's name.

In those early months I had lost one role and not found another. Others were doing for Dad what I had done. Others took my place as prime caregiver, protector, and companion. Hardest of all was finding my role of confidante usurped by Mae. Dad and Mae were the new intimates, sharing their days, growing in affection and mutual knowledge. Only gradually, as I was weaned from my complete responsibility for Dad, did I rediscover my old relationships with family and friends. I progressed from the self-pitying, "Dad doesn't need me," to a somewhat relieved, "Dad can get along without me being there so much," to the final comfortable, "Dad and I are both leading new lives that serve our needs."

Over the months our relationship seemed to settle into something more like it had been before Dad's illness. Of course, I still paid the bills and monitored his care, and he grew weaker and more forgetful. But, freed from daily dependency and caregiving with all its accompanying drama and tension, we became two people who loved and enjoyed each other. The nursing home had made it possible for us to find ourselves again.

In other ways, my horizons expanded. Dad's roommate, Fred Barr, originally appeared to me as solemn and unfriendly. When I came to visit Dad, Mr. Barr would never respond to my overtures. Then, invariably, he would either wheel out of the room or turn his back on us. One day Mr. Barr motioned me to his side.

"Excuse me, Mrs. Phillips," he apologized shyly. "I am profoundly deaf and the hearing aids do little good, so please forgive me if I appear unresponsive at times. I called you over because I'm concerned about your father not getting enough rest. The night nurses whip in and out of here so fast, I don't believe they're aware of how little he sleeps. I'm a life-long catnapper myself, so I see how terribly restless and wakeful he is. I thought you should know."

This was my introduction to the way in which nursing home roommates look after each other. It was also my introduction to that kindly, interesting man, Fred Barr, who was all alone in the world. Our friendship grew to the point where I began to say quite naturally, "I'm going to the home to see Dad and Fred."

Dad's final descent began on a Monday and ended peacefully on a Thursday. My younger brother, Chris, and I were with him as were Mae and Fred—his old family and his new one. My feelings were serene as I sensed that it was time for Dad to go—time for us to release him.

At my suggestion, Fred Barr was later moved to Dad's place by the window, a choice spot for a deaf man who needed more opportunity for watching the world. Dad is gone, but I visit my close friend, Fred, every week.

And somehow, with the nursing home experience, Anne and Annie have at last merged into one person.

The personal experiences which follow, four of David's, one of a student, and two of Sally's, capture the humanness of those who live and work in nursing homes. They have been transforming experiences, much like that of Anne who discovered not only a new Dad, but a home in which the human spirit can have new meaning.

"THE BLANKET"

A gerichair is quite different from a wheelchair. To begin with, it has four small wheels instead of two big ones. The back of the chair slants at a slight angle and offers little cushion for comfort. An all-purpose tray, and sometimes a "posey strap," holds the rider firmly in place. It is best propelled by going backwards. The occupant looks much like a lobster as he or she pushes against the floor and reaches out to passersby while backing down the hall.

On this particular day I am learning all about gerichairs, pureed food, and limited mobility. It is clear that one reason for putting a resident in a gerichair is to control distance and speed. Nevertheless, I finish my pureed peas and proceed backward down the corridor at a remarkable pace.

It is quiet on the floor. Most of the residents are taking a nap and the 7-3 shift is excitedly waiting to depart as the 3-11 group is soon to arrive on the unit. I find myself very much alone at the far end of the hall when I discover two other souls breaking the code of silence.

I spot them as I pass the activity/dining room area to my right. Normally it would have been on the left, but you have to remember I'm going backwards. I slide by the entrance before finally stopping. I think I see two residents circling each other in their wheelchairs like two wild dogs in a face-off over a piece of meat. "What craziness is this?" I think.

I push my way back to the entrance for a better look. When you're in a gerichair you need to plan ahead sooner; the maneuver is not easy. Finally I peer around the edge of the door to watch the combatants. They appear disoriented and confused. One of them is an aged man whose skin drapes over outstretched bones as he makes a wide circle around a woman in the middle of the room. The lady is leaning forward about to drop out of her chair. I am reminded of the Indians closing in on Custer as I watch him move around and closer to her. And then I see the blanket.

The small, white piece of cloth is bunched up on the floor caught beneath the wheels of the woman's carriage. She cannot reach it. As I look upward into her frustrated eyes, I see for the first time the reason for her anxious and embarrassed state. Her leg has been amputated and without the blanket her stub protrudes like a diving board over a swimming pool. Her nursing home gown covers little as she is sitting on most of it from the effort to reach the blanket. She is practically naked from the lap down.

The humanness of the man suddenly becomes clear. Instead of closing in for the kill, he is making attempt after attempt to reach the woman's cover. With each pass he stretches until his arthritis can take it no longer; it is too far away. Finally, unable to stand the frustration, and also out of my own embarrassment for failing to see this human drama acted out from the very beginning, I back into the room and join the effort to retrieve the blanket.

On the first pass I am amazed to find how much the tray and "posey strap" restrict my movement. I cannot reach it either. I know this helps the old man save face, but on the second pass I get it. I turn toward the woman whose silent cheers I can hear loudly, but at the last moment, I back up to the man and hand him the blanket.

I watch as he gracefully slides his chair across to the woman and slowly but efficiently covers what is left of her leg. She looks him directly in the eye, and says graciously, "Thank you very much." With that, she turns and leaves the room.

I realize that these were the only words spoken during the entire episode. I am exhausted. I look at the man (who, I learn later, is 106 years old), and just sit there. After a brief period of staring at each other, he begins to smile. I smile back. We know we have been humans in the midst of the leper colony.

"A SCREAMER AND A MOANER"

Nothing will unsettle the nerves more than a person in a nursing home who is a screamer and a moaner. Sally's roommate in 107A was such a person on that fateful night described in Chapter Three. Anyone in close proximity is naturally affected. Sometimes an entire floor will get caught up in the noise and tension-producing sounds emanating from the mouth of a single individual. Visitors from the outside, already uncomfortable, become terrified by the screams unless otherwise knowledgeable about such things.

Generally, my reaction to a person who yells and screams is to withdraw from the area as quickly as possible. I am not drawn to the individual; I want to escape. One day when visiting a nursing home in my clown make-up and attire, I had no choice but to confront this most dreaded situation.

I had one hour to spend on the skilled care wing. Bill Mathews ("Bags"), an authority on clowning, had taught me that clowning in a nursing home is different from performing on the street. In the home, the clown talks, touches, loves, and kisses. The white paste, symbolizing death, provides an anonymity which quickly disarms pretense and game-playing. Self-revealing stories are often exchanged in one or two visits instead of the usual eight or ten. It is phenomenal what a person will share with a clown.

I take the elevator to the top floor. Why, I wonder, is the skilled care wing always at the highest level, or furthest from the front door, or separated from the other units by bushes, shrubbery, or a driveway?

The nurse at the station can't miss me as I bounce out the door with a big grin painted across my face. Before she can respond to the change of pace, I say, "I've got 60 minutes, who needs me?"

"Olga," she replies quickly, "Room 428."

As I start down the hall, she adds, "Good luck, David, she's a screamer and a moaner."

Fear grips me and it only intensifies as I near the room. The moaning can be heard by everyone yet everyone pretends not to hear it. It is deafening to me. I want to turn around and leave, but with the paste on my face, I think I might get through it. Thus, with my true feelings disguised behind the mask, I enter Olga's room to loud grunts and groans.

Olga, a small woman, slowly rises off her bed with each extended cry. I approach her side and pull up a chair. I forget my costume and simply try to establish conversation. No response.

With the next moans, coming like labor pains now, I lean over her and ask loudly, "Olga, do you hurt?"

She reclines to a prone position and screams, "Yes . . . yes, I hurt!"

Encouraged at establishing contact, I begin again with small talk. It goes nowhere. She seems to be unaware of my presence as a person or as a clown.

Finally I stop talking and lean over her shrunken body. Catching a moment between moans, I reach up and begin tracing the wrinkles spread across her forehead. She seems to relax. I slowly caress her face. She relaxes more. I am now making love to her face with my hand. She is no longer screaming or moaning.

I continue the love-making and imagine to myself how the exciting chapters of her story might read. No longer frightening, she looks beautiful. I begin to realize that it is my attitude that made her something different from what she is. And she certainly cannot hurt me. How could I be so fearful? I like this woman very much and she hasn't even opened her eyes.

As I carefully hold her face in my hand, time races by. It is the first time in my personal and professional experience that I fully understand the power of touch. After 20 minutes, I am convinced she has fallen asleep.

With precise timing, I slowly withdraw my hand and move away from the bed. Before I can turn away, she leaps suddenly off her pillow and while I expect more screams, she says quietly, "Please don't go."

I move toward her and resume the fondling. She relaxes and settles back. This time I can sense her reliving the exciting chapters herself. She is clearly a human story in a human body in a human drama. And I think I am the performer. How wrong.

"MADISON STREET"

Mr. Campbell sits in the line-up everyday. He plays with imaginary objects on his tray and everyone treats him like he is a vegetable. All forms of communication are directed at him rather than shared with him. When he does try to put an idea together, others finish his sentences for him. He is too slow, and they are impatient.

I walk by Mr. Campbell every morning on my way to class. I always speak to those who give back some sort of response, but never to him. This particular morning I am in a hurry to get through the gauntlet so I rush by. He slaps at my thigh as I charge past.

"Hey . . . hey, Sonny!" he yells.

I come to an abrupt stop and turn to see him staring at me like a lost dog in the park. I want to be on my way but I am transfixed by his stare. He holds me for the longest time. I want to turn away but I have hesitated too long. To back off now would send a message of complete rejection. I squat beside his wheelchair and grab his outstretched hand.

"Good morning," I say.

No response. He just holds on, very tightly.

"And what is your name?" I ask.

"Campbell," he replies, looking away.

His attention is attracted elsewhere but he refuses to let go. I try again. "Where were you born Mr. Campbell?"

His head jerks toward me and he says very loudly, "Madison Street."

On a hunch, I say, "In Chicago?"

"Yes!" he yells back, "Chicago."

"I've never met anyone from Madison Street," I reply. "Isn't that the street known as skid row?"

"Yes!" he exclaims again, but this time with a smile. "I've been a bum all my life."

Our conversation is beginning to draw a crowd. Two aides, a resident sitting on the other side of Mr. Campbell, and a student arriving late for class stand in awe and fascination with the exchange that is going on. We are all amazed. This is not a vegetable. Mr. Campbell is a human being.

"A bum?" I inquire.

"Yes, a bum . . . A skid row bum . . . A bum . . . A skid row bum." He begins to drift off into memories which would probably stun the group now gathered around him.

"Do you miss it?" I try to bring him back.

"Miss what?" he asks.

"Madison Street," I reply.

A long pause. Everyone is waiting for the answer. An aide starts to answer for him. I wave her off. He is thinking.

"No. . . . I don't miss it . . . ," he starts slowly. "But I'd rather be there than here."

The reality of his response is overwhelming. Skid row is hell, but it's better than this hell. Mr. Campbell's sanity is still intact. He simply appears to be "out-of-it" because he frequently withdraws from this world into a world of his own. His vegetable-like stance in the line-up is no different than that of the young teenager who has been forced to go to church. He is in it, but not of it.

"I think I would rather be home too." I rise to my feet, squeeze his hand one last time, and add, "I must be on to my class now. I will stop and talk again tomorrow."

As I turn the corner I sneak a look back down the corridor. Mr. Campbell is still staring at me. We share something now. For a brief moment he moved out of the twilight zone, and said, "Hi, this is me."

"THE COOKIES"

Dawson almost died. He was on a respirator for nearly two weeks, in and out of two rehabilitation hospitals, and finally placed in a nursing home near his hometown. His mother died prior to his illness and having never married, his only relative was a brother who lived 500 miles away. Our church was the primary caregiver from the outside. I visited in the early "hospital" days, but now that Dawson was in the nursing home, I found myself disconnecting more and more. Worse, I could see the nursing home from the interstate every time I drove home from work. The guilt resulting from not visiting my friend regularly was beginning to haunt me.

One morning near lunchtime, I decide to leave work early in order to tend to errands I have been putting off. I am almost home when I spot the Pleasant Vista Nursing Home across the highway. I think of Dawson. The car seems to turn on its own at the exit to the home. My guilt is now driving me rather than me it. I go out of a sense of duty.

Dawson is sitting in the hallway. A magazine lies open in his lap but he is about to drift off into a different world. I startle him as I lean over too close, and probably say too loud, "Good morning, Dawson!"

He adjusts his eyes, straightens up, and says, "Well, hello, David."

Feeling the stares of others, I ask if I can push him down the hall where we can talk in the privacy of his room. He nods affirmatively.

Once in the room I recline on one of the empty beds and begin a bit of small talk. He seems interested but distanced from what I share about the church and the people in it. The Kansas City Chiefs bring less of a response. I am getting very uncomfortable. I realize I am only here out of guilt, a sense of duty, and I am anxious to be on my way. I have come to the nursing home for me, not for Dawson.

"Have you ever been out of here, Dawson?" I ask.

"What do you mean?" he replies.

Getting more courageous and honest, I say, "Well, I really didn't want to come visit today because I have several errands to run. But it would be nice to have you along while I do them. Would you like to come with me?"

"David, I haven't been out since they brought me here from the hospital. I don't think they will allow it," he answers.

"It's not a prison, Dawson. If they will let me take you, would you like to go?"

Excitement begins to dance in his eyes as he says, "I would love it."

I rush down to the nurses' station and share my plan. There is some reluctance since Dawson is incontinent, but I assure the staff that I can handle everything. They agree, and I sign him out.

Getting the wheelchair into the trunk is more difficult than transferring Dawson into the car; it takes 20 minutes. Nevertheless, we get aboard and begin our trek around town. He is wide awake.

I drive to the bank, the local utilities office, and renew my automotive vehicle license at the appropriate bureau. Dawson waits in the car while I do my business. The car wash is especially fun. He sits quietly inside while I spray the windows and soap the whitewalls. We go for a drive through the countryside in our clean car and I point out some of the damage caused by a recent storm. He enjoys it all.

We have been gone for two hours, the errands are finished, so I say to Dawson, "It's time to go back. Is there any last place you would like to go before returning?"

"Yes, could we go to a grocery store?" he asks.

"What do you want to get?" I respond trying to buy time to think of a reason why we shouldn't go.

"Cookies, I would like to get some cookies," he says with conviction.

Not thinking of any reason why not, I agree to it. We find a rather large store, and while it takes another 20 minutes to get him unloaded, we accomplish the task together.

Several persons in the store are astonished to see Dawson. It is clear they have had him dead for some time. They are particularly embarrassed at what to say. None have visited him since he moved to the nursing home. I just stand back and watch them struggle with their conversations. Others are surprised to see us there as well. I guess seeing an incontinent "patient" from a local nursing home in the grocery store is quite a sight. Nevertheless, we move on through the rows.

The cookie section spreads across several shelves. Dawson takes his time as he surveys the possibilities. Finally he selects several kinds and we load them on his chair (not a bad substitute for a grocery basket). We work our way through the check-out counter and proceed to the car. It takes only ten minutes to get on our way this time. I am getting better.

It gets real quiet in the car. I wonder if Dawson is fatigued or sad to be returning. We are nearly there when another reason suddenly comes to mind as I reflect on Dawson's silence. "Dawson," I ask, "you're not supposed to have the cookies, are you?"

The long pause is a sufficient answer. Furthermore, Dawson has never lied in his life. Finally, he replies, "No."

I think hard and fast. After a long span of more silence, I say, "Well, I guess that means we will have to sneak them in!"

"Yes!" he comes to life with renewed excitement.

We both feel like Jack Nicholson in "One Flew Over the Cuckoo's Nest" as we make our plan to sneak the cookies past the nurses' station.

The strategy works perfectly. I carefully keep the full attention of the nurse behind the desk as I sign Dawson in. He, in turn, leans over the cookies tucked beneath the blanket on his lap. After passing the guard, we move quickly down the corridor to his room.

Before I can say good-bye, he urges me to help him hide them. "We need to stash them several places. That way if they find one batch, I will have others," he explains. Hiding the cookies is an exciting climax to an enjoyable afternoon.

Taking leave is not easy. I share with Dawson how enjoyable the day has been. I review how it was that I didn't want to visit, yet, as it turns out, it has been just great. I haven't laughed so hard in a long time. I thank him for all of this, and add, "And next time, Dawson, I will know what to bring you . . . and we can hide every batch."

To my horror, Dawson begins to cry. Tears flow down his cheeks, but he is able to hold back the sobs. A sensitive but tough man, it is obvious that he rarely cries in the presence of others. We are both suddenly uncomfortable. I reach out and hold his hand. "What is it, Dawson?"

"David . . . It has been a great day for me too. . . . It was fun going all over town. . . . But I don't want any cookies. . . . All I want is your fellowship. . . ." We embrace as tears flow everywhere.

A sense of belonging, of participating, of being part of some sort of intimate relationship, brings drama to life. Dawson has brought it to mine. He has taught me how to be human.

"MY FRIEND MARY"

Ruth Olmsted, one of our students and also a nurses' aide in a local nursing home, shared this story:

"'We care' it said in big black letters on the red badge I wore pinned to the white uniform. They had finally given me the name tag after 3 1/2 weeks as an aide at the Greenlawn Care Center. It was a routine night. Working the 3-11 shift was easier than the mornings. Things moved a little slower and quieter. Supper was over and I had been working at putting people to bed.

"Each one required the same routine: take off clothes, wash face, hands, bottom, lotion back, put on gown, help into bed, rails up, lights off, good night. I had done it dozens of times.

"I had left Mary for last that night. She was always so uncooperative—hitting and pulling at her clothes to try to keep them on. I was in a pretty good mood. I didn't want to ruin it. But the time had come when I had all the others in bed. It was time to 'do' Mary.

"As usual, I found her clear at the other end of the hall scooting along in her gerichair. Because it had no foot rest, she always tried to stop forward motion by dragging her feet. I found that pulling her from the back was the easiest way to move her. I grabbed hold and started down the hall dragging Mary behind me."

"'Don't go that way!' she shouted. I stopped abruptly. Mary seldom put together three words let alone a comprehensible sentence. I looked back at her, turned the chair around, and pushed from behind. To my surprise Mary held her feet up and did not try to stop our motion.

"'That's good, Mary. I'll put you to bed now,' I said wondering if she really did understand. But as I passed another wheelchair Mary grabbed the hall railing and stopped our progress. Just as I thought. She wasn't talking to me at all. She was probably talking to some nonexistent someone known only in her mind. It must have been a coincidence that she said it at the same time I started to pull her chair. I grabbed her hand and pried it off the railing. When I finally got it loose, she grabbed hold of my hand. Not feeling like fighting her to get my hand back, I just put it up on her shoulder and began pushing her down the hall again. I placed my other hand on her other shoulder and she grabbed it too.

"When we got to her room, she let go of me. I turned on the light and began to prepare the bed. As I worked, I started to sing 'You are my Sunshine.'

"'I like that song.' My God, it was Mary again. I spun around in my tracks and stared at her.

"'What did you say Mary?' No answer. 'Mary do you know that song?' No answer. I sat down on the bed looking straight at her in the chair and began to sing again. 'You are my sunshine' . . . echo 'sunshine.' 'My only sunshine' . . . Again an echo, 'sunshine.' Mary was singing. She didn't get many of the words, only a few in echo, but hummed along in tune. We continued singing as I got her ready for bed. She didn't fight to keep her clothes on or resist my washing her at all.

"When I had her in bed, the song was over. I was pulling the covers up when both of her hands shot up toward me. 'Oh, here it comes,' I thought. I should have known this was all a dream. You can't put Mary to bed without being hit at least once.

"A hand landed on each side of my face but instead of striking they simply held on tightly and pulled me down. She pulled herself up and kissed me on the forehead. 'I love you,' she whispered.

"My eyes full of tears and a lump in my throat the size of a basketball, I bent over and kissed her forehead. 'I love you too Mary,' I said through my tears — now flowing freely down my cheeks.

"She touched my cheek with her hand. 'Friend?' she said in a questioning voice.

"'Oh, yes, Mary. We are good friends.' She leaned back and closed her eyes. I whispered good night as I turned off the light.

"Once in the hall I spotted another nurses' aide coming out of a room. I started to tell her excitedly about Mary. 'Jan, Mary . . .'

"'I know, can't she be a bearcat to put to bed? She hit me three times last night when I was undressing her. She kicked Betty in the stomach yesterday morning.'

"'She's my friend,' I replied as I started down the hall.''

The humanness that resides within each of us can reach out and zap us at anytime.

"THE FEAST"

When I was in David's "The World of Nursing Homes" class, he admonished students visiting in the facilities to "go into a room you'd rather be shot than enter." I found my room the first day.

About all I could see was white sheets. But at the top was a head—a death's head, I thought to myself. The skin was stretched so tautly over the bone, it more nearly resembled the skull it would become than the head it now was.

I forced my feet to move; I forced my hand to take her hand— more veins than flesh. The eyes flew open, and I froze.

"Honey," she shouted, "I never felt so awful in my whole life!"

Unable to match her honesty, I muttered sympathetic, banal platitudes. Never mind, she was deaf.

"Tend to me, Honey!" she ordered.

Befuddled, I began some ineffectual bits of pillow fluffing and sheet tugging.

She raised her head, shaking it in disgust, and announced, "It's not enough!"

And it wasn't. But she was. I was hopelessly in love with this wild old lady, my Gabby. A friendship had begun that would come to its physical end only when I committed her body to the ground four years later.

In my sentimental ignorance, I had thought she was dying when we met. My class journal reflects this. It also reflects that what I was really dealing with was a determined 88-year-old lady who was beginning to recover from her stroke.

On my second visit, I found Gabby pulling herself up by the bedrail with her good arm and declaring, "See what I'm doing, Honey? Well, it's what I want to do."

Several weeks later, after the tubes had been removed and the pureed food exchanged for a soft diet, she commanded, "Get me some Kentucky Fried, Honey!"

Gourmets often discuss what they call their most "memorable

meals." For Gabby and me, this was a memorable meal in the human sense. Our feast was spread out on the tray of her gerichair. We used humankind's original silverware—our fingers. Our dinner music was made up of our sighs of satisfaction and purrs of pleasure. Gabby herself pronounced the blessing through a grease-anointed smile, "Honey, this is the best meal I ever ate!"

Food remained for us a tie that bound and allowed for mutual giving and caring. We broke many rules, medically and nutritionally, but the nursing home staff accepted the reality of Gabby. Her room was her home and meals were for sharing. She shared her tray with me and I brought in hotdogs and endless bread and butter (mostly butter) sandwiches for her.

Gabby never accepted therapy after her stroke. She saw it as "hurtful" and fought the therapists. As a result, the affected arm and hand remained useless and her legs grew more and more contracted. One of the cancers which regularly appeared on her face began to spread, eventually covering her left eye. But she still liked to eat. "Get the recipe for that, Honey, it's good," she'd say.

At the end of Gabby's journey, my feeding of her became our chief way of communicating and loving. The staffs of the nursing home and the hospital, sensitive to our need, were kind and helpful. Gabby was still in charge, taking or refusing as she wanted. I was still "tending to," more or less awkwardly.

I think I sensed that our last meal together was just that. Each bite given and taken was an act of love.

For four years, Gabby and I had shared a feast of laughter and love—a human feast.

"LOST AND FOUND"

Together we had been through three different nursing home placements and one attempt to "make it" again in her own home. Though I was not her "blood kin," emotionally I had become Marion's family. We had shared her increasingly unmanageable temper with all its humiliations, and her severely failing memory with its embarrassments and anxieties. But, we had shared good moments, too — companionable outings and projects, quiet times of thoughts, laughter, and memories.

Even as her legs weakened and the wheelchair became her day-time home, Marion seemed to drift away. Eventually, I wondered if she was "in there" at all. When I came on Sunday, I would regale her with everything in the week which I thought had even a remote chance of entertaining or amusing. No response — only a "nobody's home" stare.

Desperate one Sunday, I grabbed one of her old, well-worn books. Much had been lost during the moves, but two important items remained — Marion's favorite book and her little black velvet hat without which no respectable Episcopal lady of Marion's generation could function.

The Shenandoah was marked and underlined in places. I knew that it covered the Civil War, a passion of Marion's. Whenever we would pass by the park where a battle of that war had been fought, she would say, with tears in her eyes, "I can always hear the Boys in Blue when I'm here."

I opened the book at random and began reading an underlined section describing the beauty of the Shenandoah Valley. Looking up, I saw to my utter astonishment and joy, tears streaming down Marion's cheeks.

"Marion," I exclaimed, "you're in there! This is a place you loved, isn't it?"

"Yes," she whispered.

Quickly, I located another marked passage — a humorous story about a general attending a Sunday church service. As I read, she chuckled, really chuckled.

That was all. She would make no comments and answer no more questions, but she was there, her heart and her humor still intact.

The Sunday before Marion died, I found her comfortably settled in her old wing chair. "I couldn't bear to put her in the wheelchair any more," said the nurse.

To my surprise, Marion's little black hat lay on the nearby table. Why was it out?

As I sat with Marion, anticipating the deep sadness for me and the relief for her that death would soon bring, the young cleaning girl came into the room.

Pointing to Marion's hat, she said, "The other girls and I put it on her yesterday. It was wonderful! We could see what a handsome, dignified lady she is."

You were in there, Marion. The girls and I found you.

Chapter Eight

Discoveries

In the theater of life, most of us choose to ignore the exit signs. Having made our entrance, we believe we will want to stay on indefinitely.

There are few places that remind us more forcefully that there is a required exit for each of us than the nursing home. Worse, the nursing home shouts to us in ear-splitting tones that our exit may not be easy or pretty. Our natural instinct is to avoid the whole thing, hoping that we will be one of the lucky ones who die at a ripe old age blessed with physical competence and mental alertness. The suggestion that we face up to aging and death sounds like the grim admonition of a masochistic schoolteacher.

Yet, as we have stated earlier, we discovered that the only sure-fire cure for the fear of aging and death is to embrace the enemy. Immersion in the apparent ugliness of the nursing home enabled us to discover its beauty. Had we surrendered to our natural desire for escape and avoidance, our fears and apprehensions would have been forever riveted in our hearts and minds.

Sometimes we found gold nuggets among the pebbles — incidents and knowledge that revealed the beautiful nature of nursing home life and its people. At other times, we discovered life-saving paths that taught us how others had found their way in the wilderness. We learned new ways of looking and listening, and new ways of interpreting what we saw and heard. And finally, we learned new ways of responding. With acceptance, love of nursing home life was born.

This chapter is perhaps one of the most important segments of our book. Here we share quite honestly and humbly, our experiences with the human spirit. We have learned to put our own agendas aside and to let the residents themselves teach us about life and living in the final phase.

PHYSICAL IMAGES

David

Several years ago I was invited to deliver a keynote address titled: "Celebrating the Strengths of Aging." It was an experience I will never forget. It went like this:

A bit nervous at the prospect of facing an audience of 2,000 persons, I paced back and forth in my hotel room like a caged tiger. The butterflies would not go away. To ease the tension I turned on the television and settled restlessly onto the bed. As my mind drifted from opening statement to opening statement, the TV suddenly grabbed my attention.

"They call these age spots," a gracious elderly lady was proclaiming as she pulled back the sleeve of her blouse. "I call them ugly," she continued.

The commercial, promoting a well-known hand cream, filled the remaining 50 seconds with claims that the product would fade away the processes of aging. I was beside myself. Here I was, preparing to celebrate the strengths of aging before a large audience, and this woman was telling millions of Americans that "aging is ugly." While it provided material for my opening remarks, it clearly reflected negative images of aging and further reinforced societal fears and anxieties about the changing appearance of the human body.

Changing skin, sore bones, unpredictable plumbing, and diminished reflexes are indeed concomitant signs of the aging process. The lady advertising the skin cream, however, would lead us to believe that these changes are not inevitable or natural. In fact, the corporation she represents would like to claim that aging is even preventable. What nonsense. But people believe it. They want to believe it.

Fears of physical deterioration are particularly enhanced every time a person walks into a nursing home. For many it confirms all of their worst anticipations. We began this book by exploring the "leper colony" because *this* is what people see when they come through the doors.

What I discover when I visit a nursing home is something different. Where I once saw lepers, I now see beautiful, unpretentious human beings. Stripped of societal creams which enable people to put on synthetic smiles and fabricated faces, these precious individuals show depth and reveal meanings unaltered by cosmetics.

They are forced into a presentation of self without the use of normal props. Makeup will not cover arthritic limbs, and legs requiring wheels inevitably force the drama to a lower level. But the more I interact with these persons, whose costumes give away the secrets of the backstage, the more I admire their performances. They are real.

If the audience, visitors, and other performers in the drama can get beyond the "physical" curtain, they will discover a setting painted by human hands, not stagehands. And it is beautiful.

Sally

For a number of years I worked as a volunteer with handicapped children, many of whom suffered from the body-distorting effects of cerebral palsy. One of my favorites was a sharp and witty boy whose crippled legs were of little practical value, but he put them to use as instruments of fun and humor. His favorite trick was to grab one of my legs in a scissors hold, usually catching me unawares as I passed by. He was a tease and we both enjoyed it. I recall one day wiping some wayward food off of his shins and realizing I loved those scarecrow legs. Body and personality had become one.

It was the same in the nursing home. Hands with veins like miniature mountain ranges patted me with affection and reached out to be held — and I loved them. Legs propelled toward me like a marionette's manipulated by a drunken puppeteer — and I loved them. A voice warped by stroke uttered unintelligible words of concern for a roommate — and I loved that too.

The grandsons of a woman whose funeral I was to conduct greeted me at the mortuary door saying with youthful zest, "Go look at Grandma. She looks just like she did before her stroke!" They were happy with the smoothed out wrinkles and filled out cheeks—the idealized face of an idealized better time; I loved the road map of living that her face had become. The odd walk, the lolling head, the chorus of words repeated again and again become objects of affection when they are part of a known human being.

When we are young, we may have a list of desirable physical qualities we seek in a lover. But after years of loving someone, are we really sure which is the cart and which is the horse or which came first? Do I love your smile because it is beautiful or is your smile beautiful because I love you?

I worked intimately with people in the nursing home when I was chaplain. One day I realized I had become a fan of the aged human torso. Unexposed to the elements, there is a kind of innocence and simplicity about this area between the lower neck and upper thighs. The loss of firmness and muscle which we all dread, seems instead to be a natural relaxation of the flesh, which, having achieved its purpose, rests in a different kind of beauty.

In my home I have several vases of treasured dried weeds, plucked from the fields just before they died. As they aged, the weeds turned brown—wonderful shades of brown, no two alike. It seems to me that weeds, like human beings, have two particular times of beauty—at their fresh, tender beginning and at their mature, worn ending.

Beauty is indeed in the eye of the beholder. But the eye is educated by the mind and heart. In the nursing home, our eyes can be reeducated if our minds and hearts are open to new ways of looking at and beholding human beings.

THE LINE-UP

David

We have said much about the "line-up," yet its ubiquitous presence in nursing homes deserves further comment. Nurses' aides are unsure as to why they "line them up," and even residents themselves say little about it.

Our hunch is that space has much to do with it. There are very few open areas in nursing homes and tension runs high as space diminishes. When animals of any sort are confined to such overcrowded conditions all kinds of reverberations are set in motion. Consider your own uncomfortable reactions when someone you don't know penetrates your personal space. While this is addressed in our section on privacy, it has relevance here as well.

The next time you are seated in a theater-like arrangement—with both chairs facing forward—try carrying on a conversation with the person at your side. After a time your neck will begin to ache and your eyes will strain against their sockets. A natural invisible barrier is erected between you and the other.

And so it is in nursing home line-ups. All attention is focused into the center of the corridor. Residents are spared staring at each other and do not feel obliged to engage in forced conversation. Thus in spite of overcrowding, a bit of privacy is carved out of the otherwise tense climate.

Most rooms are semiprivate. Space is at a premium here. Questions of turf become an issue whether or not residents specifically mention it. The caregivers seem to sense a need for dividing territory and as a result often create "mini-line-ups" in the rooms. So instead of facing your roommate, opening possibilities for interaction, you sit staring at a dresser, out the window, or into the hall. Conversation under these circumstances becomes directed to those who enter the room, not to the occupant who shares this little world with you.

The way space and distance are negotiated by staff and residents may be one reason for the development of staff-resident relationships and the relative absence of resident-resident relationships. All activity, even in most activity programs, is focused toward a specific other who usually holds a position of authority. Rewards (and punishment), then, get exchanged with staff rather than with residents. Sociologists have shown for years that social structure has a direct influence on human behavior. This is as true in nursing homes as it is outside of them.

While line-ups may be advantageous to residents who seek privacy in the midst of openness, I have discovered that by wheeling my wheelchair around to face them, conversation is facilitated and natural. It is appreciated more than resented, and those with whom I have shared stories are grateful.

I feel it is important for visitors in nursing homes, and for staff as well, not to hesitate to disrupt the line-up. In fact, a commotion on one end of the line will draw the attention of others — everyone gets involved. Boldness to refuse to accept things the way they are is a useful trait for persons living, visiting, and working in the world of nursing homes. Shyness will get you nowhere. It will also prevent you from discovering the human colony.

Sally

My first extended encounter of the day in the nursing home was a visit with the first floor line-up. They sat there in their wheelchairs in one of the choice spots of the house; it was in an extension of the lobby hallway and just a stone's throw from the first floor elevators. This was the Grand Central Station of the home where everyone would pass by sooner or later.

As though going to work, residents Marie, Ethel, Marguerite, and Verleater, headed for the line-up after breakfast. Each had her place and each had her role. I, too, had my role. Every morning I would (1) kiss Marie on the cheek and we would talk, (2) kiss Ethel more formally (she had an innate dignity and reserve) and we would talk, (3) touch Marguerite and we would talk, and, (4) kiss Verleater on the mouth and we would kid and carry on. Thus blessed and stimulated by the line-up, I would head for my office with a light heart and an eagerness for what lay ahead.

One area where you always find an established line-up is near the nurses' station. LPNs with paperwork and phoning responsibilities develop close relationships with line-up residents. In fact, this is sometimes the most fertile ground for LPN-resident friendship. No matter what else she is doing, an LPN will have a subconscious alertness to what is going on in the line-up. Was that a low moan from Ida who hasn't been feeling well? Nurses become equally adept at tuning out the fussers and chronic complainers. With sensitivity, a resident who is unusually restless and/or confused will be taken into the station itself for safekeeping. The staff tells the story of Elnora, who, with all the nurses away for the moment, answered the floor phone and said to a startled caller, "They've all gone. I'm the only one left."

As Chaplain, I viewed the line-up as both a help and a hindrance to my work. On the positive side, it allowed me to meet and talk with some people every day. On the negative side, I could rarely talk with them privately. Our relationships could be loving but somewhat superficial. One lesson I learned quickly — if a resident in the line-up wanted me to pray with them, it was their need against my self-consciousness about praying aloud in such a public place. It was no contest; I quickly lost my self-consciousness.

People assume roles in the line-up. One may be a comedian, responded to and appreciated by his or her fellows. Almost always, there is a caretaker alert to the others' needs and quick to summon nurses for help. The time spent together in the line-up may appear to be of little social consequence to the uninitiated, but, in reality, close and caring relationships are born and nurtured.

I recall visiting Marie, a regular in the line-up, when she was taken from the home for a brief stay in the hospital. I returned to report on my visit, and while Ethel, also a regular, did not respond when I spoke of Marie by name, she got very excited and interested when I explained that Marie was the lady who always sat next to her. The name had escaped her, but the person was known and loved.

The line-up, perhaps more than any other nursing home phenomenon, points up the need for staff, family, and visitors to understand its dynamics. What we see is only a shadow of what is happening.

WAITING

David

In nearly every nursing home there is space which serves as a "dayroom" for those who would like to sit quietly, watch TV, look out the window, listen to music, read, or just wait. Very often it is at the end of a corridor or conveniently situated in a central spot with architecturally pleasant surroundings. Included in this social space are plants, usually artificial ones. Some dayrooms are carpeted. Made to look like a family room or den, this area is designed to be appealing, comfortable, and away from the hustle and bustle of the home. The only problem is it is empty most of the time.

Few people congregate in the dayroom. It is simply not where the action is. Residents in a nursing home can be found bunched together at major intersections, in the lobby, and along well traveled corridors. Staying in the dayroom would rob them of variety, excitement, and new faces and personalities. The brain, stimulated for a lifetime with new information, loses power when it is no longer challenged to engage and respond to new cues. And the best source of stimulation comes into the nursing home from the outside. No wonder we feel like we are "on stage" as we walk through the gauntlet. We represent new blood, new life, new possibilities.

Looking at residents sitting in the line-up may be depressing to those who venture into the nursing home infrequently. Their thoughts may trick them into thinking that the residents are just sitting there waiting to die, when in fact, they are sitting there looking for some excitement in an otherwise ordinary day. If they wanted to die, they would stay in their rooms and completely withdraw from self and others. No, those in the line-up, the lobby, the intersections, and the corridors are looking for something to happen. The mind is still working.

Even residents who have trouble remembering what day it is, or who they are (and especially who *you* are), can find a more interesting existence out in the halls. The next time you find yourself in a nursing home, stop by a lonely old soul and visit for a while. Don't worry if the person confuses you with friends, relatives, and/or caregivers. Just visit. Don't worry if the response is not what you want or expect it to be. Your presence is what counts. And for those starved for conversation, have patience. Listen and love. Be of service. Sometimes a resident can sit there for hours, like a hitchhiker waiting on the side of the road, before some kind person stops to give them a ride.

Sally and I discover fantastic things about the human spirit by stopping to say "Hello in there." What is rewarding about this effort is the discovery that the residents end up being of service to us rather than the other way around. Their stories and images are full of life and imagination. They fill you with hope, not despair. The key, we have learned, is to put our own agenda aside. It is not important that specific information about the past or plans for the future be accurate. If the images are real to the resident then they are real enough. What happens during these encounters is the combining of energy sources to produce a different reality than what existed before. Life becomes shared.

Waiting for a meal, a bath (or shower), a doctor, a nurse, or a friend to visit builds up a sense of anticipation in the resident. Some will organize an entire day around an anticipated ten-minute visit from an outsider. And what is wonderful is that even after the visitor has gone, the resident will continue to think and talk about the nice person who came to visit.

Nonambulatory residents who spend much time flat on their backs respond to and anticipate visits as well. Looking forward to being turned in the bed, getting a pill, anticipating a change in shift (new caregivers on the floor), and a meal in the room can bring excitement into the day. It is absolutely amazing how little it takes to help a person deprived of attention to feel better. Sally and I, in our own lives, have come to appreciate the little things too. We may have learned it from the humans in the leper colony.

Sally

When we can no longer do some things for ourselves, we must wait for others to come and do them for us. Most of us will put off that day for as long as we can.

An older person who doesn't drive or has given it up will seek housing in a place where shops are within walking or busing distance. Another will move from his or her home to an apartment because, "I can no longer keep up with a big place, but I can manage a few rooms." Self-determination and control of one's activities are natural and normal human goals. They may not be the divine ones.

Sooner or later, as we grow older, most of us end up waiting. We wait for the daughter or the daughter-in-law to take us to the store, the doctor's, the beauty or barber shop. We wait for the son to come and help us fill out papers. We wait for the grandchildren to visit. We wait for the neighbor to come change the light bulb, repair the faucet, or mow the lawn. We wait for family members to get home from work and telephone us. Waiting is a new skill which demands of us a psychological adjustment as well as a physical one.

The nursing home may be the place we go for an unwanted advanced course in the art of waiting. New methods and attitudes must be learned. Some persons develop wonderfully assertive skills that combine their remaining resources with those of designated helpers. I knew many such people in the nursing home. For every skill they lost, they found an alternative way of doing what they wanted or needed to do. If one were to list some of the accomplishments of old age, this creative flexibility would surely be one of them. Even during the short 24 hours that David and I wore the mantle of nursing home residents, we discovered the beginnings of this adroitness in ourselves.

Eventually, however, time and deterioration may have their way with us. The physical skills that spelled success for the wheelchair-bound won't suffice for the bedridden. Flexibility and adroitness are no match for incontinence. When we reach this state, all the negative forces of old age seem to cry out, "Gotcha!" When this happens, attitudes, not skills, make the difference, a bedridden, incontinent expert once told me.

I had come to visit and found her in a soiled bed. She had been waiting for help for some time, so I went to look for a nurse. When my friend had been restored to some degree of comfort and dignity, I returned. Dismissing the intended purpose of my visit, I drew up a chair and asked humbly, "How do you manage it?"

She smiled.

"Let me tell you first about how I *didn't* manage it," she confided. "I used to lie here in a mental state far worse than the physical discomfort of a wet bottom. I would see myself forced to lie helplessly waiting for others to come take care of me. I was eaten up with false pride, resentment, and self-pity—and my anger at God would have destroyed a lesser deity!

"To make myself feel better, I thought about all of the diapers I had changed when I worked in a nursery school. At first, that just made me feel that, by gosh, I had earned my right to some help!

"But then one day it occurred to me that while I hadn't been fond of soiled diapers, I had been fond of soiled kids. Somehow I'd forgotten to separate these two facts. The nurse disliked cleaning up the mess therefore the nurse must dislike me. As unpleasant as the waiting for help was, it was really my negative feelings about myself that were causing my depression. So I screwed up my courage and began to talk to the aides about it.

"They were wonderfully frank and open with me. One admitted she hated days when she had four incontinents to care for . . . 'but, Honey,' she said to me, 'shit is shit and people are people. I never get the two mixed up.'

"Another one said, 'If it rains on my picnic, I don't blame the clouds. It's not something *you* do, it's something that just happens.'

"The aide I'd worried the most about told me, 'When I'm cleaning you up, I'm seeing myself in this bed someday — and I'm going to treat you just as I want to be treated when my time comes.'"

My friend smiled again. "I don't like to wait, but I wait easier now that I feel O.K. about myself and them. It's enough," she said.

Not good, but good enough.

TIME

David

Along the lifecourse there are periods when you have too little time and other periods when you have too much. In a nursing home there is never enough time for staff, and for residents there is too much time. But it does get organized in a number and variety of ways.

Outsiders, during brief visits to a nursing home, may see only idleness, boredom, and despair among residents sitting in rows or lying in beds waiting to die. This, in turn, leads to discouragement for the visitor who feels perplexed about what to say or what to do. Worse still, when not visiting, the outsider's image of their loved one is of a person suffering from aloneness, depression, and feelings of abandonment. Time passes so slowly that family members find themselves wishing for it all to end soon. This heightens feelings of guilt.

What the visitor misses is the busy schedule of meals, baths, activity programs, people-watching, and the drama surrounding bowel movements. There is much around which to organize one's day. We are all waiting to die, but some of us are in the meantime occupied with survival. This is true in a nursing home.

One day I saw a lady sitting on a patio in her wheelchair all alone. She looked terribly depressed, lonely, and bored. After some struggle, I managed to get my wheelchair out the door and joined her there.

"Pretty day," I said as I opened what I hoped would be a conversation.

"Yes," she replied softly. She seemed in a different world. Staring into space, she did not bother to look at me. I sensed in her a desire to talk.

"My name is David. I am visiting here today."

She turned in my direction but remained detached. She said nothing.

"I guess it can get boring and lonely here sometimes." I wanted so much to let her know that I understood some of her pain and misery, and I was giving her a chance to talk about it.

She turned toward me so suddenly I was startled, "Young man," she began, "do you feel the breeze on your arm?" She lifted her arm as a sign for me to do the same. I, of course, immediately did so.

"Do you feel it?" she asked again.

"Why, yes, I do," I responded.

"Doesn't it feel good?" she inquired.

Feeling like I was losing control of this conversation, I replied, "Yes, it does feel good."

"And do you feel the rays of the sun on your body?" she continued.

I again followed her example by turning my face and limbs toward the sun, and without a doubt, the rays did feel good.

"They feel good too," I said honestly.

We both just sat there for a while. It was like two persons watching a spectacular sunset and to talk would be blasphemy. I had been so preoccupied with my images of her loneliness, I never realized how beautiful the day was. And now I, too, was getting lost in reverie.

"Bored you say?" She sliced into the serenity with complete

disregard for the communion we had established. "Young man, I just love it out here!"

Time is a personal affair. Residents spend it in different ways. I have learned not to make judgments about what may appear to be boredom, loneliness, and depression. What is important is to say, "Hello in there."

Crossing the threshold from being an outsider to an insider is accomplished by spending *more time* in a nursing home. Visits at mealtime, during activity programs, and in the morning, afternoon, and night will provide a better sense of what the world of the nursing home resident is like. Unfortunately, time is more of a problem for the visitor than for the residents.

Sally

Older people, when we listen to them, give us a glimpse of how it will be when we reach their age. I have heard many older folks say that hours and days go slowly, whereas the weeks, months, and years go by with alarming speed. Time is bound to look different to one who knows his or her own time is limited by a definite number of years.

During my tenure in the nursing home, I never heard a bedridden older person complain about time. Others complained for them— "Mother has been sick such a long time." I have felt that same pity myself. But I never heard an older person put it that way. My conclusions about this are mere speculation, but I surmise that as immediate memory diminishes and yesterday's memories grow more vivid, the present becomes less real and therefore, less troublesome. There may be many blessings in old age which are hidden from the young and middle aged, and unsung by the elderly. We need to listen, and then listen some more.

Older people often have a sense of time that is real and important to them—that is, a sense of when it is time for them to go, to die. I once jumped aboard an emergency ambulance that was taking a 99-year-old resident to the hospital. Every modern, sophisticated device was being employed to keep her alive. Knowing her as I did— knowing that she had been yearning to die for a long time—I begged the paramedics to cease their efforts. They wouldn't, of course, and one of them later said to me, "Lady, nine or 90, I want them to live." Thus speaks the system. But, humanness won the day; my friend died in spite of their efforts.

I recently visited another lady who had failed almost beyond recognition since I had last seen her. She lifted her head up, and looking at me with clear eyes, said, "It is time for me to go home." This is the time message we need to understand. When the aged know it is time to go, we must not hold on to them.

MEALS

David

As stated earlier in this book, a meal is not a nutritional event. It is much more. The federal nutrition program initiated over a decade ago learned this in its infancy state. While there is indeed a direct correlation between nutrition and health, nutrition site managers and others quickly realized that participants in the program came to the site not for the meal, but primarily for the fellowship.

Widows and widowers find mealtime the most difficult adjustment to the survivor role. Mealtime is special. The holiday feast shared by family members is recorded on film, in diaries, and stored away in memories for years to come. It is a ritual, a symbol, a time for renewal, an occasion to remember the past, enjoy the present, and contemplate the future. And most of us experience it as enjoyable all along the lifecourse.

In nursing homes, meals are somehow different. They seem to have less significance socially, but new rituals prevail. For example, while residents are not often seen chatting and carrying on conversations in the dining room, there is always a stir if someone sits in the wrong place. And people notice if meals are not delivered in a particular order. A ritual is followed, but the litany is one of procedure, not celebration. A careful study of mealtimes will reveal some interesting dramas.

Watching an adult child feed his or her 98-year-old grandparent will move anyone to tears if watched long enough. Only a few residents are fed each day by a visitor, but the act of feeding the hungry and giving drink to one who thirsts is an act of affirmation with sacred overtones. The adult child's action brings back special memories to anyone who has fed or has been fed by others. All *homo sapiens* would die in their infancy if not given sustenance by someone. Many die in old age for the same reason.

A visit at mealtime is special. It is more natural to share a conversation over a meal, and the table offers a common bond which draws the visitor and the resident together. It is also an alert time. People notice who is present and who is absent. To an outsider the setting may appear grim and foreboding, but much is always going on in a nursing home dining room.

Mealtimes, like visitors, also provide an organizing element to the day. Preparation may take more time than the meal itself. Getting back to the room (if the meal is served in a central dining room) adds time as well. Passing to and from means movement and encounters with others along the way. It is like sitting in the line-up and taking one's place in the gauntlet. Where there are people gathered together, something is bound to happen.

I went to see Dawson the other day. Remember Dawson and the cookies? As the nurses' aide gathered him into his wheelchair, she asked me if I would like to join him for lunch. Although wanting to seize this moment as an excuse for exiting, I said, "Sure. . . ."

We sat directly across from each other as his meal was placed between us on the table. I immediately got into the role of feeder as the strawberries were large and Dawson could not cut them. He would never have been able to pull apart the milk carton, and the salt substitute, sealed tightly in plastic, would not have substituted for anything had I not been there. He appreciated my help, but it was my presence that he relished. A nurse could have fed him food, but I fed him fellowship.

We talked for two hours. The other residents came and left — each taking notice of our in-depth discussions of the stock market, banking, Maine, the church, and stories out of the past. We were thoroughly engrossed and oblivious to our surroundings, when a nurses' aide startled us by cleaning up the last pieces of food from the floor. The lights had even been turned off, but no one had stopped the flow of energy passing between us.

Sensing somewhat of a sigh from Dawson, I asked, "Are you tired? Do you want to go back to your room?"

"Oh, no!" he replied quickly, "I'm enjoying this chit-chat. But if you need to go, just say so." We continued for another 30 minutes.

Yesterday I took Dawson some cookies. Because of his "low sodium" diet I checked with the nurses this time. They calculated the amount he could have and I delivered them with a clear conscience. But the nurses were different on this particular day. They took more time with me. Soon it became evident why. They appreciated my spending two hours with Dawson on the previous day. It had helped them, helped Dawson, and made them less "short" on the floor that afternoon. I was going to tell them how much it helped me, but I didn't.

Sally

A saint would be hard pressed to survive the role of Director of Food Service in a large nursing home.

While the general quality of meals can be improved and perceived by most as improved, individual preferences place the food director in a "damned-whatever-you-do" position. I have sat in on resident food committee meetings and heard each person ask for the opposite of what his or her neighbor has just requested. Your idea of good potato salad or meat loaf is not mine.

Furthermore, reason is in short supply here. A few sensible souls may accept the fact that institutional food, by its nature, has certain limitations. But most of us find it hard to be reasonable about food when, in a less active existence, it becomes a focus of our day.

I recall one gentleman who took drastic action after a month of receiving white toast when he had asked for whole wheat. Each morning he would simply pick up the offending bread and drop it on the floor. He was roundly tut-tutted for his actions, but he won his battle. I admired his spunk. Sweetness and mildness do not accomplish much under such circumstances. Individuals in nursing homes may well need to learn new tactics to get what they need and want, particularly at mealtimes.

As David has observed, the whole process of sharing a meal is rich in its implications of humanness. One woman who had come to the nursing home with great reluctance and regret confessed to me,

"I had forgotten during all those years of living alone and liking it what fun it is to share meals. I am so eager now to get to breakfast to see how Shirley and Marie have fared during the night. When I went to the hospital, it was what I missed the most."

I have written of how food and feeding became the way in which Gabby and I expressed our mutual love. In the nursing home where I worked, there were two men, a son and a grandson, who arrived daily to feed lunch to their loved ones. Because of their loyalty in this act of daily feeding, each of these men maintained a close relationship with his mother or grandmother. Inevitably, they adopted all the other people at their table into their noontime family, thereby extending the blessing of their practical help and personal support to other residents and staff. *Their* tables "came alive."

When we were short-staffed on a heavy feeder floor, I would sometimes ask the aides to assign someone to me to feed lunch. There is no questioning the fact that such an act deepens one's knowledge of another person and creates closeness. This is particularly rewarding when the resident has lost many of his or her communicating skills and is therefore often ignored or overlooked.

I had an experience as Chaplain that was particularly painful and points up the need for greater understanding of nursing home problems and residents' needs.

Vera was having many difficulties with eating and required more time and attention than the staff could realistically give her. I was thrilled when I remembered that above Vera's bed was a large note declaring that the included list of names were her church group members who wanted to be called if there was anything she needed. I chose the president's name, phoned her, and explained Vera's and the staff's problems. I suggested that some of her church friends might be willing to come regularly at lunch or dinner to feed her, thereby giving them an opportunity to visit as well as give Vera the help she so sorely needed.

To my total astonishment, this Christian woman expressed herself as outraged that the nursing home would try to "drag in" friends to do what the nursing home was being *paid* to do for Vera. So offended was the lady that she followed up with a call to the nursing home director to "report" me and complain further about my request.

Perhaps I had done a poor job of explaining, but even with a good explanation, I suspect many people would have had a similar if less violent reaction. We assume or want to believe that money will cover nursing home residents' needs. It will not. And even if it did cover the basic ones, it would not supply the deeper human needs of our friends and family. Only we can do that. There is no better example of this than mealtime.

PRIVACY

David

As illustrated in Chapter Three, the world of the nursing home looks very different from the vantage point of a wheelchair. Not only do you see more, you can often observe others without their knowing it. I think it is the angle of the eyes and the sitting position. You are like a camera on a tripod—you can turn away in an instant yet maintain a steady stance.

What I enjoy most about being in a wheelchair is the immediate feeling of closeness with the residents. Not only do I feel drawn to them, I feel accepted by them as well. We share something that no "outsider" could possibly experience unless he or she, too, takes on the vulnerable position.

What is most discouraging is to have persons penetrate your personal space without an informal or formal invitation. Each one of us, whether in a wheelchair or not, has a private zone surrounding our person which, when violated, makes us very uncomfortable. This is particularly the case when the intruder is a stranger. If you are not confined in a wheelchair you can more easily escape or withdraw, but if you must confront others from a sitting and compromising position, turning away is much more difficult. In short, there is little privacy. You find people, often strangers, coming right up to your side, leaning over like a tree frozen in an ice storm, asking you a hundred questions. They always get too close, making any chance of a social bond negligible.

The need for physical distance is often accomplished psychologically. I have found that by turning away and saying nothing the intruder's conversation will be cut short. No wonder so many nursing home residents seem to turn away or withdraw when approached boldly by staff and/or visitors. Only by spending time in wheelchairs have I discovered the importance of personal and social space.

Staring is also a form of penetrating privacy. Persons with any kind of disfigurement understand "the stare" better than anyone else. The only way to ward off the glancing and sometimes darting eyes is to look away. And it is important to look away before the stare holds you too long. If this happens, it is likely that you will see the person react. It will in all probability be negative, a grimace or a squint, or perhaps the starer will look away too. It is not a comfortable experience for either party.

The biblical account of the leper colony requires the leper to yell out "Unclean! Unclean!" to warn those approaching. Sometimes the nursing home resident would like to sound a warning as well. To avoid the uncomfortable stares it would be easier to ward off the intruder from the beginning. This is, of course, impossible. The resident is powerless to control his or her environs. Privacy becomes sacred. You find it by looking to the side, down in your lap, or by shutting your eyes.

I don't stare at nursing home residents anymore. If my glance is held too long, I realize the necessity of approaching the person for some sort of conversation or contact. It is like entering a person's house by mistake, but alas, you are discovered. The only way out is to engage the surprised occupant with an explanation. To cut and run may create suspicious thoughts. No wonder paranoia is so common in a nursing home.

Privacy involves space. And there is simply not enough of it in the world of the nursing home. Not only is the space immediately around you precious, the social space in which you move about becomes an important extension as well. It is important to respect the living environment of the resident. Each little niche can have enormous meaning. Take nothing for granted.

Sally

My office in the nursing home was in the same corridor with residents' rooms. I thought of the women across the hall from me as neighbors whose privacy I would respect; they saw me as a new intimate and drew me into their liberated version of privacy.

As reality would have it, there are days when an aide calls in sick and the work of the nursing home floor must be carried on by fewer people. This means delays. Residents who would normally be up and dressed are still lying in bed at 10:00 a.m.

Mable had her own solution to this problem. She called me into her room and announced that she could not stand another minute in bed—would I help get her up? I protested, and threw logic and reason her way. She pooh-poohed everything I said.

"I know my part and I know the nurse's part. I'll show you what to do and we'll be just fine."

I knew a superior force when I encountered it. Besides, I too, wanted her happily ensconced in her wheelchair.

We got her up and on her way. That day and in the days to come, Mable gave up her privacy to me with infinite grace and good humor. Her healthy sense of values chose being out of bed and making a new intimate over the protection of her personal privacy. Life changes and Mable changed with it.

It was not easy at times to know whose privacy was being threatened. Helen, another hall resident who was wheelchair-bound, discovered that at the time of day when she had serious and urgent bathroom business, nobody but the Chaplain was around to assist her. Again, I was pressed into service, but far more reluctantly this time. Assisting someone with a bowel movement was a greater assault on my personal privacy than transferring a resident to a wheelchair. At first, I just helped and departed as fast as I could. Then the humanness and the humor of the situation began to get to me. Helen and I developed a routine and a repartee that knocked us both out. We thought we were funny, we thought the whole process was funny. We looked forward to it—almost.

Better yet, this new intimacy enabled Helen, whose speech and side were severely impaired, to attempt to compose letters to her daughter dictated to me. Sometimes she couldn't think of the word she wanted or couldn't say it. Sometimes she could say the word and I couldn't understand it. We had more trouble than Harpo Marx, but just as much fun. I always signed the letter to Helen's daughter with the remark, "Your mother and I go to the bathroom better than we write letters.'' I hope her daughter had a sense of humor.

In Chapter Three, David and I both have related incidents when bodily privacy escaped us. On rereading these, I am fascinated to see that neither of us experienced this as loss. After a few momentary twinges of discomfort, we were both relaxed with nakedness and body functions. As David has observed, with age and nursing homes, masks are dropped and the curtain rises to reveal what has been going on backstage. The wonder of it is that it can be experienced not only as all right, but as good. It is as if the loss of our roles and our masks frees us to be fully human in spite of ourselves.

CONFIDANTS

David

What is it that makes life a drama? What makes it worth living? What makes it the exciting enterprise that it is?

If the staff and the administrators of the nursing home in which I reside have not struggled with this question, then I'm in trouble. How can they possibly care for me if they don't know what it is that makes life worth living? Unfortunately, in most nursing homes the question is rarely asked or considered. Thus, I am in trouble.

"David, let me tell you about life and drama," one lady told me. "We were in our 30s, my husband and I. We were hiking up to Loch Vale Lake in Rocky Mountain National Park . . . 2 1/2 miles from Bear Lake . . . straight up it seemed. We strayed off the trail to witness one of the most spectacular sunsets ever painted. He reached out and hugged me tight as the sun slowly rested behind the mountain. We were one with God, one with nature, and one with each other, and he never even said a word. But, oh God, I will never forget it.''

This story, and others like it, focus on intimate social relationships. Our special ties with other people make life a drama. Friendship is a complicated concept. On the one hand, we have acquaintances and friends, but as we become more intimately connected we develop close friends and confidants. The latter know our story.

They know who we are, and, in spite of knowing our secrets, they still love us. Amazing isn't it?

Close friends and confidants validate and reinforce our very being. They make life worth living. With them life is always a drama. But eventually, they die. Oh, some move away, perhaps to a retirement community, and some experience poor health which somehow changes the relationship, and for others transportation may change visiting patterns, too. But most die. The question then becomes, "what happens to us when they are gone?"

Losing close friends and confidants can lead to a psychological death long before the physical one. All of a sudden we feel like no one wants to hear our story—no one cares. We feel isolated and alone. We, too, may want to die. Why live when there is no one with whom to share our story?

One goal of Activity Directors in nursing homes is to bring people together in relationships. But it doesn't happen. In spite of being surrounded by the same people day after day, residents remain strangers.

"David, you're right about confidants," a lady told me one day, "they do make life a drama."

"Thank you," I replied, "it is something about which I feel very certain."

"Yes, but you know, I don't want any more close friends," she said.

"But why?" I inquired.

"Because I will just fall in love only to lose them. There is a lot of death around here, you know. I don't want to get too close," she explained.

Indeed, a fundamental law of life teaches us that if we risk falling in love with someone, we will, if we live long enough, eventually pay the price. Love and grief are inseparable. We cannot have one without the other. If we love someone deeply, we will grieve deeply when they are gone. A person who has never grieved has never loved.

At the age of 44, I have already lost four confidants. How many will it be by age 54 . . . 64 . . . 74 . . . etc.? My grandmother, at age 96, has lost every close friend and confidant her own age. She can no longer share the intimacies of her generation with someone else who experienced those same intimacies. She never will.

But while the intensity of relationships may not be as strong in nursing homes, the desire for a sense of belonging remains. Residents still want to be somebody. They want to be recognized and taken into account. They still want someone to listen to their story and love them in spite of it. The lust for attention in the gauntlet, the warm clasp of a hand that doesn't want to let go, a kiss blown across a room, and that all-knowing look with a twinkle in the eye, is sufficient evidence of the desire for relationships. Come close, but not too close, is the message.

What is certain is the desire to share a story with a significant other who genuinely wants to hear it. Treasures are buried in these earthen vessels waiting to be discovered. Not only that, but every time we listen to their stories, we accord them value and worth. Suddenly they count, they are somebody. And we provide opportunities for them to recall those glorious lived moments experienced with their close friends and confidants. We can celebrate and identify with the powerful meaning and energy that springs forth from these intimate encounters. To see them become animated, flushed with excitement, and full of laughter gives us hope. Nothing is more important in life than our close friends. NOTHING.

Sally

Picture a lovely wooded area that you pass regularly—a place which fills you with serenity and confidence. Picture it again, when after a year of drought, fire has transformed its beauty into a blackened wasteland. Continue to pass by regularly, saddened and depressed by its devastation, until one day, you park the car and walk over to mourn more closely. And there in the midst of the blackened stubble, you behold a green plant pushing bravely up out of the ground. The old woods are gone, but something of new life is there to comfort and give hope.

My perception of the confidant problem in old age runs parallel to this picture. Like the blackened woods, the loss of confidants is a heavy deprivation of old age. There will not be ever again, people who know us so deeply or who have loved us in spite of so much.

But there are "new green plants"; I have seen them and I have experienced them.

The dying are one example. The sharing is deep. I remember a woman whose name I cannot now recall. She came into the nursing home dying, and was gone in three days. As I sat with her, talked with her, and held her in her last moments, I gave and received a confidant kind of love and acceptance.

I picture two old ladies. They were victims of Alzheimer's disease and talked mostly nonsense as far as the rest of us were concerned. Yet each day they would walk the hallways holding hands, laughing, and talking with total mutual understanding. Not the old woods, but something.

And above all, I think of Gabby and myself. We never had a conversation of any depth because of her profound deafness. She knew almost nothing about me. Yet my feelings when I was with her had the same quality that I feel with my confidants — a feeling of total acceptance and love. Particularly during the last stage of her life, when her face cancer was rampant, there remained a quality of peace in our being together.

Picture yourself — with all confidants gone. Picture yourself in a nursing home — the last place you want to be. Picture another resident, an aide, a housekeeper, a chaplain, a therapist — a person with whom you are able to share yourself, good and bad. Picture a green plant in a burnt woodland.

REALITY-ORIENTATION

David

What is reality anyway? It basically consists of agreed-upon meanings and definitions arrived at by consensus among interacting individuals over a sustained period of time. What is real depends on what people decide is real. Anyone who strays from the consensus is considered abnormal and different. If this aberrant behavior persists, the deviant takes on labels ranging from crazy, weird, confused, and for the older person, senile.

The drive to keep people in touch with reality can be seen in nursing homes across America. Whether or not reality-orientation sessions are taken seriously by residents, the intent is to keep the residents aware of who they are and where they have been. Although the third dimension of reality—the future—is rarely included, the goal is to maintain contact with the present so the past is always in context. Volunteers often get residents to review such things as who has been President of the United States and to always be alert to the current month, day, and year.

Over the years I have come to the realization that reality in nursing homes is often something other than what everyone expects or wants it to be. Nevertheless, I now celebrate imaginative trips described by residents, and I no longer have difficulty when they call me by a different name. Living in a world of fantasy is the greatest thing many have going for them. To spend a day in your mind at the lake with the family, picnicking among the wildflowers, and sailing across the waters, is quite an adventure compared to counting the "real" 10,000 holes in the acoustical ceiling hanging in the sky above the bed. Sometimes I feel like it is a crime to "bring people back" to a world which is comparatively worse.

If reality-orientation is to be successful it must only be used one-on-one, and only with persons who have a good chance of remaining active in the nursing home or who, better still, have a chance of returning to their own home. This, of course, would require a considerably larger staff and will therefore not be the rule in most cases. In my view, a better use of time would be to encourage imaginative thinking and fantasy flings. I know of one home in Ohio that takes its residents on an imaginary fishing trip once a week. The residents never leave the home, don't use poles or bait, but always catch their limit. It is enjoyed by men and women, but it is particularly fun for the men who usually have to attend activity programs designed primarily for women.

Make-believe has always been as much fun if not more fun than reality. Humor, in fact, is especially good when it stands in the face of the expected. Maybe that is one reason clowns have been so successful in nursing homes—they get away with tricks and remind everyone that while they may be in the system, they are not of it.

Sally

How one views reality-orientation depends, in considerable measure, on whether one believes that reality is the same all along the lifecourse. Consider the differing views of what preschool children should be doing. There are those who would have toddlers reading and figuring as soon as possible—pushed, if you will. Others, believing that early childhood has its own purpose and flow, would postpone any attempt to teach such skills until later. One's determination of what is realistically appropriate depends on a number of subjective values.

Among those values are cultural ones. On a scale of relative importance, would not the various races and nationalities find many differences? And what one considers appropriate and real can vary with circumstances—many people boast that they never know the date or the day when they are on vacation.

Older people who no longer work or keep house and whose outside appointments are few, may be behaving realistically when they don't know the date. Further, if one has lived through 12 or more presidential administrations, it may demonstrate rare good sense to have lost interest in knowing the name of the current officeholder.

Flights of fancy and imagination in the elderly can be delightfully entertaining to them and to us. I have taken a few "trips" with older people myself and have thoroughly enjoyed them. Certainly, it did no one any harm.

I have talked with an older person who is definitely off the track, only to have him or her self-correct before the conversation ended. My friend, Gabby, would occasionally talk about her sister, Pearl, as though she were still alive. More often than not, Gabby would suddenly snort in disgust and say, "I'm crazier than a hoot owl! Pearl's been dead for years."

I personally believe we should go gently and cautiously into this arena. We need to be humble, sensitive, and open-minded.

My own most humbling experience concerned Bernice. She came to the nursing home terminally ill, and on the first day I went to visit her, announced, "Well, you're the last person I want to see!" As her illness progressed, she began to confuse me with some long-ago beloved and kindly neighbor with whom she was over-joyed. In that fantasy, I could be her friend and comforter. Can you imagine anyone wanting to "set her straight"?

ODD BEHAVIOR

David

It is ironic that persons want everything on the inside of nursing homes to be just like it is on the outside. They want Mom to have as "normal" a life as possible, when in fact, life in this setting is anything but normal. Mom will sleep with a stranger in her bed-room, she will eat food which is predetermined and served at spe-cific times, she will be unable to take a bath when she wants one, and her bowel movements will be observed and monitored. If she gets upset, every attempt will be made to calm her down and if she screams, or raises her voice, she will be reprimanded. Finally, she will discover that some parts of the home are "off-limits," and regardless of how many times she might try, she will be denied access to them.

If confined to the home for a long period of time, Mom may never again see a wedding, attend a funeral, be part of a baptism, and in some cases, may never again receive Holy Communion. Rites of passage marking "normal" life transitions, thus providing continuity and an organizing influence, will hold less significance, and days, months, and years may blend together so that there is no yesterday or tomorrow.

Worse still, visitors and relatives come to the home wanting Mom or Dad to be normal—to be just like she or he always was. A sad scene that gets played out in nursing homes every day is the one that finds adult children weeping in the hall or in the parking lot about how Mom or Dad didn't even know their name. They want everything to be the same, but it isn't the same.

It may seem logical to expect normal behavior from an individual living in a normal environment but it is, in my experience, too much to expect it from a person who lives in an abnormal one. Indeed, maintaining "sanity" is always described as the most difficult task by persons who have been incarcerated or held against their will for extended periods. As for nursing homes, they are last on a long list of preferred living arrangements. People do not usually go there willingly.

The solution to all this is not an easy one, but once accomplished, it is a liberating force in one's life. I learned it from the residents. They have taught me to accept them as they are, not as they were or hope to be. Stripped of pretense they can only present themselves as they are today.

If we place too many expectations on residents to live up to our standards, we will keep them in a depressed state forever. Instead, we need to accept them on their own terms, not ours. What may appear to be "odd" behavior may be very "normal" in the world of the nursing home.

Sally

In the "About the Authors" section of this book, I quote a favorite anthropologist, Colin Turnbull, on odd behavior. He asserts that a particular behavior loses its oddness when we know the reason behind it. He is speaking of cultural differences, but it applies equally well to the seeming oddities which age can bring. Beyond the fact that the nursing home symbolizes for us frailty and mortality, a primary fear of nursing home visiting is the encounter with that frightening phenomenon, odd behavior.

No one in the nursing home had the power to disturb and frighten me as Ruth did. A gaunt, large-boned woman, she sat in the third floor dining room in her gerichair. Her sparse hair was pulled tautly back from her face making her spotlight eyes even more prominent. I describe her eyes as spotlights because they appeared large and high voltage, and they swept the room as though seeking out a victim. I did not want to be her victim, but as chaplain, I could not ignore her.

Approaching her with fear, my nightmare came alive. Ruth fixed the spotlight eyes upon me and said, "Go to hell, you son-of-a-bitch!" I turned and fled.

But, I could not forget her. And I could not forget that I was the Chaplain and there to serve her. So I regrouped my fears into more manageable form and began to develop ways of maintaining contact with her. I would ask her if she wanted something to drink—water or juice. It would be an exaggeration to say she expressed pleasure, but she did say "yes" and almost always accepted my offering. With courage born of desperation, I began to respond to Ruth's "go to hell" commands with "I don't want to go to hell, Ruth!" And something did change. When giving her command, she would become taut and rigid; in response to my "I don't want to go to hell," she relaxed. I began to relax a little, too.

One day I said to her, "Ruth, do you really want me to go to hell?"

"No," she replied, relaxing from her tension. Some days her answer would be "yes," but we had broken a barrier—we had communicated. She did not always want me to go to hell.

Inspired, I checked Ruth's chart and found, along with the name of her out-of-town nephew, the phone number of a friend. I have often found that old friends and neighbors can fill out the background of an elderly person who is virtually without close family. The woman apologized for not visiting, but explained that she herself was frail and old. She told me that Ruth had lived with her widowed sister and that the two together had raised her beloved nephew. Ruth had been a hard-working seamstress.

One day Ruth was not in her place in the dining room. Staff informed me they had kept her in bed because she did not seem well. In bed, Ruth looked more vulnerable—as we all do. But, she rose off of the pillow in her usual rigid way and I braced for her usual greeting. Instead she said, "I want to go to Louisville." It took only a second for me to recall that Louisville was where her nephew lived.

"You want to go visit your nephew, is that it, Ruth?"

"Yes," she said, relaxing back on the pillow.

I explained that she was not really well enough to travel such a far distance.

She turned and looked at me and my heart almost stopped. Her eyes were clear and viewing me with intelligence. "I love you," Ruth said. We hugged and kissed and I told Ruth I loved her, too. A few seconds later, the spotlight eyes had returned. But I had found the real Ruth. I knew she was there.

Ruth was a great teacher. She taught me to *assume* that underneath any odd behavior, there is a real person. That knowledge enables me to approach people I would formerly have avoided. I feel anticipation. I feel hope.

Sometimes, nurses who work intimately with odd behavior will make a stab at explaining it. But more often, acceptance is the only attitude that is helpful. Finding a human being behind a frightening facade reminds us that the humanness is *always* there — whether we find it or not.

HUMOR

David

One of the last places people expect to experience humor is in a nursing home. For years now, however, I have wanted to write a book on nothing but the humor found there. Every day produces something new.

I am *not* referring, of course, to the "sick jokes" that always abound among those who work in the midst of suffering and pain. Ambulance drivers, emergency room personnel, firefighters, and police who confront misery on a daily basis often cope with the grim realities of their work by telling jokes and making fun of those for whom they provide assistance and care. This happens in nursing homes, too. Though the laughter is not vicious, it is sometimes necessary if one is to avoid crying.

I am speaking instead of real humor — the spontaneous kind that rocks you back on your feet causing you to stumble or fall before regaining balance. Ask anyone who works in a nursing home about some of the funniest things that have happened during the course of their work and they will keep you rolling on the floor.

Two years ago I was teaching a class in a nursing home and was assigning 20 students in wheelchairs to various locations throughout the home. A middle-aged, but prematurely gray-haired student showed up late. I had one wheelchair left, but I had no assignment for him.

"Go wherever you want, Alex," I said. "Discover this place. Immerse yourself and experience it as if you were a resident."

"I'm on my way." He stroked the wheels and headed down the corridor.

Managing the elevator by talking a visitor into pushing the buttons, Alex ended up on the fourth floor—the skilled care wing. He was stopped in his tracks as he passed the dayroom. There, lined up in a row, were six or seven residents sitting almost motionless in their chairs. Alex rolled into the room, made a wide circle, and joined the line-up. He slowly folded his arms in his lap and sat in a catatonic position for what seemed like hours.

Actually, only ten minutes had passed when a lady entered the room. She was bringing the Holy Eucharist to those who wanted it. The elements had been blessed at her local church by the pastor, and she was now prepared to complete the Communion Service by sharing it in the dayroom. It was her first time on the floor.

As she entered the room, she walked immediately to the first person on the end of the line-up, Alex.

"Hello!" she said loudly. First-time visitors always raise their voices. They speak to residents as if they were all deaf. These exchanges remind me of Americans who upon meeting persons of other nationalities, always speak slowly and carefully articulate or mouth their words so the foreigners can understand. That is, fully expecting them to have trouble with English, they treat them as if they were also illiterate. Nursing home residents are particularly vulnerable to such unfounded images and stereotypes. Visitors assume that they are deaf and treat them as if they were dumb as well.

Alex, fully into his role now, gradually looked up and replied softly, "Hello."

"And what is your name?" she asked loudly and slowly as she carefully articulated the words.

"My name is Alex Horvath."

"That's nice, Alex," the words were now turning into sickening sweetness clearly exceeding the normal parameters of kindness. "And how long have you been here in the home?" she continued.

"I have been here only this morning. I am a student at Saint Paul School of Theology," Alex said clearly and honestly.

As her sweet smile turned to a sympathetic one, she leaned over Alex carefully patting him on the back, and said, "Sure you are!"

Instead of arguing, "But I am!" Alex settled back in his chair and waited as she celebrated the Holy Eucharist with him.

Very funny, but sad too. Obviously the visitor had already made up her mind about Alex. She had labeled him confused and disoriented like all the rest. He never had a chance.

So it is with most humor in nursing homes. Every moment which spontaneously produces a belly laugh has a counter-reaction as well. The reality of the home ultimately sets in. But humor, in the meantime, has served its purpose — a respite into humanness in an otherwise fabricated world.

Sally

There were large floor to ceiling windows in the lobby entrance of the nursing home where I worked. It was a popular place for those looking for action and those who simply wanted to watch people come and go.

As I approached the door each morning, I would frequently spot a resident friend sitting near the window and we would go into our acts. He/she might wave extravagantly and blow kisses; I often danced a brief jig. On cold winter days I would shiver and stomp; he/she would respond with expressions of mock pity and beckon me in. One gentleman and I had a flirtation scene worthy of light opera. A day in a nursing home can be shot through with humor.

I have often thought of writing an essay on Americans and their wheelchairs. The latter, it seems to me, become an extension of our love affair with the automobile. We love our "wheels." We feel good when we are "driving" them. Maybe that's why so much nursing home humor seems to center on the wheelchair. David and I often show a wonderfully satirical film on nursing home life which features a ne'er-do-well resident who hooks his cane on the wheelchair in front of him, forcing that poor soul to give him a free ride, all unawares.

Bob was a charming man of 102. He was very deaf, smelled wonderfully of aftershave lotion, and was a delight to know. Every day Bob would take his exercise walking behind his wheelchair which he used for support. He would do the "grand tour" of the first-floor hallways. One day, coming toward each other, we fell into one of those routines where each one moves to the same side and neither can pass. Suddenly, as though struck by the same thought-lightning, we went into a matador/bull contest complete with "olés." Thereafter, we "fought" whenever we met. If you have never had a bullfight with a 100-year-old, I recommend it.

A lady whose wheelchair exercise also took her on a morning cruise down the hall, stopped me one day and commanded, "Sit in the chair and I'll give you a ride. You can pretend you're the Queen of England." It was an offer I couldn't refuse, so down the hall we went with the Chaplain-queen bestowing a regal wave to startled and amused staff and residents.

One day I was helping a lady find her address book. She had to make an important call and could not remember the number. We looked in all the right places such as her pocketbook and table drawers. Suddenly, she grabbed my hand and exclaimed, "Help me out of this chair and look under the pillow I'm sitting on!" I did so and there were her address book and all the rest of her important papers. "That's where I keep them," she said, beaming with pleasure at her own good sense.

In the wheelchair, in the dining and bedrooms, and in the bathroom, surrounded by all the wonderful raw material of humor, nursing home laughter is created from the human capacity to "think funny."

One beloved floor favorite, Verleater, met the diminishing of each of her faculties with high good humor. I would find her dozing over the remains of her breakfast. Coming awake, she would ask, "Babe, have I eaten?"

"It looks like you have," I'd reply.

"Well, by God, I hope I enjoyed it! I don't remember a thing!"

Then she would throw back her head and laugh at the absurdity of it all.

Most nursing home staff members could tell of "bits of business" or routines which they and some of the residents have developed together. My own favorite concerns my friend, Gabby, and her favorite aide, a tall, gangly young man of 19. Sometimes Jerome would come into her room, dash to her bed, let down the side rail, and climb in bed beside her—all in a split second and before she knew what was happening. Laughing and protesting, Gabby would hit at him with her good hand.

"Aren't you going to let me stay?" Jerome would beg piteously. "I'm tired. I need to rest."

It was so wonderfully ludicrous that Gabby and I were always reduced to tears and weakness, those fruits of a laughter binge.

The two places I worked where I laughed the most were the nursery for handicapped children and the nursing home. In both places, it seemed as though the worst had happened, and we had discovered that instead of destroying us, it had uncovered the best of our humanness. So we laughed.

PURPOSE IN LIVING

David

The most dreaded statement in long-term health care is heard when a "new admit" says, "I wanna go home." Or worse, when a resident of many months says, "I'm going home today," when everyone knows that no one is going home.

Over the years I have heard any number of responses to these statements. Here is a sample:

— "Now Mother, I know you will like it here. Give it a chance."
— "But Dad, you know you can't care for yourself at home. You'll be here just for a little while—just long enough to get your strength back."
— "Mom, you have been so lonely at home, but here you will have a lot of friends."
— "Why Dad, at least you will get some good food. And three meals a day too. And don't worry, I will visit often."
— "Mom, as soon as you get well, we will get you back home."
— "Dad, I really envy you. Look at all these women you have here. What a lucky guy you are."
— "They say it takes a little time to get adjusted, but everyone loves it after they've been here a while."

—"Now you're not going home just yet, but maybe someday you will."

—"Now be quiet, I don't want to hear that kind of talk."

—"Want to go home? Don't you like me? You mean you want to leave me?"

These replies only serve to further isolate the soon-to-be-abandoned person. They tell the anxious individual that no one is listening, that no one understands, and that no one cares. No response at all would be better than these.

Yet there are no enemies here. Most persons are truly crushed when asked by residents to be taken home. They just don't know how to respond. They know that they too would want to go home. After all, there is no reason to be living in a nursing home is there? There is no purpose served. Well, is there?

Sally and I think there is. Nursing home residents have taught us how to accept our limitations and press on. They have shown us how to accept rejection. They have demonstrated to us real courage. They have especially been role models on how to be patient and kind. They have revealed to us that humor, even in the midst of pain and suffering, lasts a lifetime. And they have loved us.

More than this, the residents do the same thing for all those who live and work in the nursing home. As stated earlier in this book, high among the satisfactions that caregivers experience in their work are the relationships they share with the residents. You may be able to keep your distance from patients if you serve as professional staff in a hospital, but in a nursing home you get attached to those for whom you care. And the caring is a two-way street. Many residents look forward to each day for they will be in contact with many lives—certainly more people than if they were alone in their own home.

When first entering a nursing home these realities are neither evident nor anticipated. Home sweet home never looked better. Wanting to go home after many months is not so strange either. There are many times when I would like to go back in time, too.

So what do you say to a person who says, "I wanna go home"?

You say, "You want to go home? . . . You miss home?

. . . Home must mean a great deal to you. . . . Tell me about your home.''

Then you wait to hear the whole story—all about home and how much it is missed and is going to be missed. When all is said and done, you say something like, ''Oh yes, I can see why you want to go home. It sure is a special place for you. I'm so sorry you have to be here. This can never be like your home. But I will be here with you. Let's make the best of it.'' A big long hug and a kiss will provide some additional assurance.

This kind of response lets the resident know that someone else understands. Suddenly he or she is not alone. In time, a new world of relationships begins to unfold.

Sally

Most of us on the sundown side of 40 have known times of purposelessness in our lives. These times are usually triggered by some form of loss. A loved one dies. We lose a job. Circumstances force a move to a new place. A long sought-after goal proves to be unreachable by the route we have been traveling. We have then passed into the darkened tunnel of lethargy, ennui, and depression. We have plodded on, occasionally peering ahead through the blackness to see if there was a hint of light at the other end. And for most of us, thankfully, the end of the tunnel has appeared.

Admittance to the nursing home may be the nethermost place in the lifecourse because it is the culmination of so many other losses. Loved ones and friends have died depriving us of emotional and physical support. Strength and health have diminished to the point where we cannot even hold onto or maintain what we have. Though few people have the courage to admit the thought to their consciousness, this leaving of home means one has no home to return to— ever. Previously, trips to the hospital and convalescent unit held the near certain promise of the return home. The move to the nursing home is final.

Nursing home staff will testify that those who handle this life crisis the best are those who make the decision for themselves. To look at oneself honestly, to recognize that one can no longer care for oneself, to decide not to engage others in the ever-increasing caregiver role, is itself an act of self-esteem. This is not to say that those who make their own decision do not enter into the tunnel, but rather that the light at the end is visible to them from the beginning. Working their way out may take time, but they will make it.

The elderly most at risk are those who are "put into" the nursing home. Son flies in while Mother is ill and he and her doctor conclude—perhaps quite correctly—that she can no longer live alone. As Mother is too sick to participate, Son takes charge of closing up the apartment, disposing of or keeping possessions, and selecting a nursing home. Mother is handed the decision—purchased, wrapped, and tied. Son returns home. Several months later, Mother "comes to" one day and realizes that her home is gone forever— that she has no place to return to. She enters that tunnel familiar to the nursing home staff who have witnessed this process so often. The staff and other residents will be her light, assisting her through the tunnel. With such help, most do make it.

What most people discover is that the purposes that made life worth living outside the nursing home are the same purposes that make life worth living inside the home. Self-esteem continues to be highest in those who take as much responsibility for their own care and happiness as possible. Residents who make friends with staff, who treat those who serve them as fellow human beings, discover they have a new family. Those who are willing to risk the hurt of further loss and reach out to other residents, create for themselves and others, friendship and support.

I recall a small group of "dependables" who attended every memorial service I held in honor of those who had died during the previous month. They came to celebrate the lives of their fellow residents, to nurture their own faith, and to comfort others. They came to support me in what they believed was an important act. You could almost pick them out as people of purpose by the way they drove their wheelchairs.

I remember standing with a tearful aide as she washed and dressed a bedridden woman. Between sobs, the aide poured out her story. Suddenly, the woman in the bed grabbed her arm and said, "My dear, when I was 40, my only son and grandson were killed in an automobile accident. I thought life was over—but it wasn't. I did smile again and you will too!" Purpose is all around us if we are alert to it.

I was called on to perform my first and second funerals on the same day. The morning one was a suicide death in a staff member's family; the afternoon funeral was for the resident whose daughter had refused her body. Feeling the heaviness of the load, I sought comfort when I returned to the nursing home between services. And my comforter? A woman dying of cancer. She gave me the sustaining food I needed.

Older people, filled with a lifetime of experience and the wisdom that comes from reflection on those experiences, have treasures to give us. In the nursing home they are surrounded by people who can and do receive those gifts.

A special friend of mine went through a very low period after she came to the home. One day her minister said to her, "Phyllis, you wouldn't be here if God didn't have a purpose for you." Thus inspired, she began to look around for that purpose and found it. She is an oasis of humor and common sense. She gives and receives with grace. She works with people who are weighted down in negatives, rejoicing in their positive steps, accepting their limitations. She confesses that she did not begin to grow in some ways *until* she came to the nursing home. Here, at last, is the time and the arena and the maturity to study and reflect on life and faith. Phyllis is an inspiration to me and the embodiment of the promise that ". . . the best is yet to be."

DEATH AND DYING

David

"Where is she? Grace, I'm asking you a question . . . Where is she?"

"Where's who?" Grace glanced over her shoulder as Mary pulled at her uniform.

"You know who. I always take Mrs. Cunningham this cola when I come on shift, but I can't find her anywhere. And someone else is in her bed. Did she go home?"

"Mary, sit down." As Grace turned to get a chair her mind was racing. How was she going to tell Mary about Mrs. Cunningham's death. This was going to be Mary's first experience with losing a resident. Worse yet, Mary and Mrs. Cunningham had become intimates. Mary, now 22, had grown up in a number and variety of foster homes and had only recently become a nursing assistant. In just a short time Mrs. Cunningham had become Mary's new mother. Both looked forward to the cola that Mary faithfully delivered each day at 3:15. Now Mrs. Cunningham was dead and gone.

"Mary," Grace started slowly, "I have some bad news. . . ." Before she could continue, Mary was up on her feet and on her way to the restroom. Tears dropped on the floor as she closed the door with a sound that clearly forbade anyone to follow. Grace just watched and prayed.

As she waited for Mary to collect herself, Grace realized how little privacy there was for staff to "let go" emotions which so often had to be suppressed. Losing a resident with whom a loving and positive relationship had been established was particularly difficult. Especially for a new aide, and especially for Mary who craved love and who had found it from Mrs. Cunningham.

Ten minutes passed. No Mary. Grace rearranged a few things at the nurses' station and decided to approach the restroom. Just as she reached the door, it opened.

Mary's face was red. What little makeup she had been wearing was gone. Braids of hair were stuck to each side of her face where she had attempted to wash up. She took Grace's hand and they walked into the empty room across the hall.

"When did she die?" Mary asked quietly.

"She died early this morning. The ambulance was leaving when I came on shift at 7:00. I think the report said she was having difficulty breathing around 5:00 a.m. The doctor was called and he told them to get her to the hospital. Everyone I saw said she was dead before she left."

"Did she go peacefully?" Mary wanted more information.

"I think so. She . . ."

"Grace, Mary, what are you doing in there?" It was the charge nurse.

"I'm telling Mary all about Mrs. Cunningham," Grace tried to explain to the agitated nurse.

"Well, we don't have time around here for little chit-chats. We have six people to get cleaned up and dinners to deliver. Get busy!" The command left little doubt that compassion, caring, and coping with loss would have to wait.

Grace started out the door.

"Why didn't anyone call or tell me about it?" Mary still wanted answers.

"They don't know how much we love some of these people, Mary. They only care about keeping the families informed, getting the body out of here, and filling the bed to maintain the census." Now Grace was mad.

"I thought this was a caring place when I took the job," Mary said.

"Me too!" Grace responded as their pace quickened as they approached the shower area.

Mary stopped Grace, held her two arms against her side and said, "I loved her you know."

"I know," Grace responded.

"And she loved me too," Mary continued.

"I know she did," Grace said in an affirming tone.

"Hurry up!" came the booming voice.

Mary began crying again as she prepared the tub for the next occupant.

By now word was getting around that Mary was taking the death pretty hard. The Director of Nurses, tired from her eight hour day, decided to talk to Mary before leaving the home. She spotted her in the shower stalls waiting for another resident.

"Mary, could I talk to you for a moment?" she asked politely.

Not knowing what to expect, Mary joined her in the hall.

"Mary, I know Mrs. Cunningham's death is a big blow to you," she began, "but I must remind you that you are to take a professional stance toward our patients. You can't allow yourself to get so close. . . ."

"But she loved me," Mary protested.

"Yes, but you can't afford to love them back. It will interfere with your work. A lot of people die here and if we have to stop and grieve every time it happens, no work will get done."

"Yes ma'am," Mary answered with dejection.

"Now Mary, don't get upset. You're young and you have very little education. When you've worked here longer you will learn how to be more professional and less personal. I know, I had to learn, too." The Director gave her a symbolic hug, patted her on the back, and told her to have a good evening.

As she walked away, Mary watched. She stared down the corridor until the boss was out of sight. Grace returned with a resident and Mary followed them into the shower room.

"What did 'Lady Charming' have to say?" Grace asked.

"Oh, nothing," Mary replied.

"Oh, come on, what did she say?" Grace knew the rest of the staff would want the details of this meeting. "Lady Charming" didn't come onto the floor to comfort staff all that often.

"She said I shouldn't get so close to the patients," Mary answered. "But the bitch doesn't know that the only person who loved me in the whole wide world was Mrs. Cunningham," she cried. "She said I was dumb and needed more education. She said I was too young to understand. She told me to have a 'good evening,'" Mary mimicked the Director's voice.

"It's so easy for her," Grace responded, "she just sits on her ass in her office all day."

"Yeah, and she's full of shit, too." Mary was really into it now. She was finally grieving.

While this little drama was getting played out, the resident waiting to be bathed was all ears. As Grace and Mary lifted her onto the lift, she looked them both in the eye and said, "She's full of shit all right . . . yes, indeed . . . she's full of shit." She grabbed Mary's arm and added, "Honey, I will miss Mrs. Cunningham, too. I know how you feel. God bless you."

Sally

One of the questions most frequently asked of me when I worked in the nursing home was, "Isn't it terribly depressing being around so much death?" In fact, the opposite was true. I have never felt more comfortable with death than I did during those three years. I knew fully the truth of the dying old woman's statement to her nephew, "When you reach my age you will understand that death is as necessary as sleep." This could be discussed endlessly in theological, philosophical, and sociological terms, but suffice it to say for me, that my own sense of its truth grew out of experience with death in its natural order and place.

When one reaches 50, there will be at least as many loved ones among the dead as there are among the living. This factor increases in direct proportion to age. I recall the sensible words of a woman to whom I had been sent by a nurse concerned about her lack of will to live. The woman said to me, "I thought I wanted to see my great-granddaughter grow up, but it just doesn't seem that important anymore." She was not depressed; she simply felt she had experienced enough. She was ready to go, to move on.

Expressing a welcoming attitude toward death is difficult to do in front of families and caretakers. Sometimes, the chaplain was the only safe person with whom to share such thoughts. I, in return, received the gift of openness and naturalness. Once residents had told me how they really felt about death and found that I was comfortable with it, they could begin to live in my presence. I treasure the memory of Crystal's funeral. There in the cemetery amidst the fields of a small Missouri town, I could at last share with Crystal's family the wonderful gallantry and humor of her last days. And they could laugh and be proud.

Each funeral, each death, has its own special meaning to me — but none more special than Marie's because the service was held in the nursing home. No one would have attended Marie's funeral had it been done at the mortuary — family and friends were gone. But the nursing home, her new family, did her proud. Housekeeping cleaned and polished in preparation. The Activity Director volunteered to sing. During the hour before the service, busy staff members came briefly to pay their respects. Marie's corridor turned out in mass — some of them people who never attended any kind of in-house function. They seemed to be comforted by the sight of Marie, who had spent so much strained effort in breathing, peaceful at last. When I finished the service, each resident spontaneously came up to me and we embraced. We had been Marie's family, and we knew it.

As Chaplain, I learned many wonderful lessons in humility. I saw faith manifested in the suffering old woman who waited serenely in the conviction that God would give her no more than she could bear. I saw the same faith manifested differently in those who refused further treatment because they were "ready to go." I ceased to be opinionated on such subjects as open caskets, coming instead to respect the individual needs of those who mourned. Death is a great humbler.

I have held the dying and kept watch with them. I can only say that there is in death the same wonder that is in birth. A life beginning and a lived-life ending are at opposite ends of the spectrum, but each is a natural part of the whole. The sense of mystery, the sense of all creatures being as one, touches every witness. Experiencing this is part of the reward of working in a nursing home.

Chapter Nine

A New Vision

"I'm going to report that place to the State Health Department!" the self-appointed advocate begins. "The conditions are deplorable. Every time I go to see Mother I have to pass by all those vegetables sitting in their urine."

"With this new survey we can really nail them for violating the rights of patients," an inspector gloats with a gleam in her eye.

"Our office is committed to protecting the dignity of all persons who live in our 200 nursing homes across the state," a state director claims.

"We are forming a committee to take our grievances to the nursing home Board. Will you join us?" a guilty family member tries to coerce others into action.

Advocacy, taking a stand, has its place in American society. What often happens, however, is an all out attack on the party or organization viewed as the perpetrator of evil deeds. Legislation and/or some sort of reform may follow, but bitterness and divisions of loyalty remain.

While we view this book as a statement of advocacy, we want to make it perfectly clear that our approach is of a different kind. We wish to affirm nursing homes and the love and conflict which resides within them. We are not against them, we are for them. And our objective is not to attack from the outside looking in, but rather to invite the outsider to join us in witnessing the story that resides within. Insiders are important, too. We wish to take their experiences as the basis for imaging the nursing home in new and exciting ways. Ironically, both those on the outside looking in, and those on the inside looking out, are often blind to the drama that is occurring before their eyes. On their behalf we want to put it in a new perspective.

We are not like the advocates who demand reform, nor like the designers and architects who have as a goal the covering up of what exists there. Instead, we hope for a change in attitude, a change in spirit, a change in commitment. Every nursing home in America cannot compete with the luxury homes that are being constructed for the affluent but frail older persons of this country, but every home *can* experience a new excitement, a new sense of meaning, and new directions as we move into the 21st century.

In one of our nursing home classes, we used four different facilities as teaching centers. One was a church affiliated home, attractive in building and grounds with many physical amenities and a feeling of "gracious living." Another was a for-profit facility, also well-appointed with the space and activities one expects in such places. The third was a converted mansion with tree-shaded grounds, which, though not built with the needs of the aged in mind, was nevertheless appealing in its feeling of openness and light. The fourth home was in the inner city — two large, old homes connected by a covered walkway. Here, there were *no* amenities of a physical nature. It was rundown, worn-out, and crowded. Yet, when David put the question to the class and to ourselves, "If you had to go to a home tomorrow, which one would you choose?" the majority, including ourselves, chose the inner city home. We backtracked as we thought of space and privacy limitations and lack of activities, but our spontaneous, gut-level choice had been for the home where humanness reached out and enveloped us.

Homes of the future, if they are to do more than simply treat and maintain the physical presence of persons in the final phase of life, must begin to look beyond the exterior person and appreciate and accept the internal humanness asking to be seen and set free. Honesty, acceptance, relationships, and play need to replace pretense, distance, disconnectedness, and professional services. People are not pieces of machinery to be oiled and cleaned; they are beautiful stories and testaments to what life and living is all about. In this last chapter we want to share with you more of what we have discovered by saying to them and their caregivers, "Hello in there!"

HONESTY

Pretense is the name of the game. Another word for it would be dishonesty. Too much pretending goes on in nursing homes and a bit more honesty could go a long way toward improving things. As we all know, when small children enter a nursing home all kinds of reverberations are likely to occur. The residents become more excited and alertness seems to reach new levels. What a joy it is to have these younger ones running up and down the halls. One reason they are liked so much is the fact that they are so honest. Art Linkletter once said, "Kids say the darndest things." Well, they do.

"Ma'am, what is that tube stuck up your body?" a small child asks.

Delighted that the obvious is not being ignored, the lady responds, "Why child, that's my pee."

"Your pee!" exclaims the boy as he rushes to get his pal, Janet. "Janet, Janet, come look at this woman's pee."

Innocence is refreshing. Children are unabashedly human. Could it be that true personhood is only revealed at opposite ends of the life-cycle? Perhaps, but most certainly during the middle part of life synthetic smiles and fabricated faces get exchanged between the actors. This can particularly be the case in nursing homes.

Sweetness, for example, can become intolerable. While a kind and loving manner is indeed an exemplary form of behavior, when forced it becomes condescending and coddling. After a lifetime, people get to be experts at picking out the frauds. A sincere voice, patience, and a genuine desire to listen can be easily detected. The sage can discern who is playing a game and who is not.

A glance at the faces of nursing home residents who are forced into group activity, forced into having fun, is evidence enough of what happens to recipients of planned happiness. Resident response to the King and Queen of Hearts Party described in Chapter Three captures some of the consequences of forced fun. Residents look away or down into their laps, and since there is no chance of escape, the response is to withdraw psychologically.

We talk child-like to those in the infancy of life, and we do the same to those in the twilight years. While the manner in which we address the child may under some circumstances be understandable, the same treatment accorded an older person is misplaced, inappropriate, and sad. There is something to say for maturity. We may not except it from the child, but we must always anticipate it from the adult.

> "Turn over the board!" the elderly lady requested of the nurse.
> "Turn over the board?" the nurse inquired.
> "Yes, turn it over," the sage requested again.
> "Honey," the nurse responded, "there aren't any boards in this room. Now go to sleep."
> "Well," the older woman replied with a sigh of indignity, "sometimes they are called pillows."

Aware of subtle interaction rituals and of gaps between the generations, some long-term care facilities and corporate bodies insist on a "professional stance" toward *all* residents. While professionalism has its place, we do not feel that the human spirit wishes to close out its existence in a sterile atmosphere of professional robots whose care is limited to what is listed in a job description. If caring is the goal, total personalities must be given the freedom to interact with all the gusto and uniqueness which has brought them to this place and time. In-service training for nursing home personnel should be committed primarily to human relations. Anything short of this places the focus on matters which are less essential to quality living. Some day, state and federal regulatory agencies will elevate the human dimension while maintaining their stance on quality physical care. If not, older persons will demand it.

ACCEPTANCE

Physical aging (biological aging) begins in late adolescence and continues uninterrupted for a lifetime. The body shrinks, the lungs hold less air, the heart circulates blood which flows unevenly, the kidneys process decreasing amounts of fluid, and the bones fail to resorb calcium in adequate quantities. There are, of course, many other changes. What is certain is the fact that all of our bodies deteriorate. All living things die.

The inevitability of death must be faced openly, and expected as part of life. Many people begrudgingly accommodate it while inwardly, and sometimes overtly, they are in full-scale rebellion against it. One of the favorite sayings of these folks is, "Old age is hell!" If they are elderly themselves, they will usually challenge a younger audience with, "You can't understand, but just you wait until it happens to you." These people view aging and death as cruel jokes, mistakes, depressing interruptions in what had been an otherwise good party. They will live with the process given the alternative, and they may even become reconciled to it, but they will never be accepting of nor in harmony with their own or others' aging and death. While we may not like it, we believe aging and death are part of the natural order of things.

Doctors, ministers, family members, staff personnel, and others who come into contact with persons in the final phase of life want to make them well again. They want them to be like they were. What is desperately needed, however, is for all of us *to learn to accept them the way they are*.

Our own experience has shown that freed from the debilitating effects of avoidance and fear, we can acknowledge the positive humanity of all aged folk whatever their condition. We can approach the person in the bed or the wheelchair—still aware of the bobbing head and drooling mouth—but anticipating the human being who is in there. We can acknowledge people wherever they are. If someone tells us they are going to die soon, we will not enter into the conventional avoidance game by saying, "Oh, you're just having a bad day. You'll be with us a long time yet!" Instead, we accept what the person says at face value, believing in it legitimacy and wanting to enter into the other's thinking with an openness of heart and mind. Each of us knows when we have truly communicated with another: it is when we have fully accepted who our friend is and what he or she has conveyed to us. Enrichment of life in the nursing home is totally dependent on staff and visitors who can do this.

As life grows more basic, humor becomes the oil that lubricates the wheels. People can bemoan memory loss as a tragedy or like

Verleater and her forgotten breakfast, see it as the comedy it is. Not taking ourselves so seriously is the perfect attitude for the final act of life. The elderly and those who love them and work with them are daily confronted with the choice of crying in despair or laughing in acceptance.

Acceptance is symbolized for us in the words "urine" and "pee." Urine is a word that goes with "specimen"; pee is a word that goes with "pants." The former is a medical and laboratory word, an avoidance word that pairs with "smells of. . . ." The latter is a family and friend word, an acceptance word that pairs with "I've gotta. . . ." If you are still urinating rather than peeing, we suspect you have not quite accepted your humanity. Do so before you grow another day older!

RELATIONSHIPS

"Give me just one person that I can look forward to seeing each day and I will be just fine. If, on the other hand, there is no one I want to see, let me die." Arthur looked forward to seeing Sally each day and Peggy on Monday evenings. He wanted to live.

We begin life in relationship with other persons. In fact, our very survival depends on it. Life in the final phase is no different. The will to live is severely tested when we feel that we have nothing to live for. And in old age, nothing means nobody. As we near the end, we become acutely aware that we will not take our possessions with us, and when our confinement disconnects us from nature (the great outdoors), we have only others from which to draw strength and energy.

While many persons outside of nursing homes have the attitude that, "that is where you go to be forgotten," they fail to realize that true abandonment occurs when no one cares to listen to your story and you don't care to listen to their story either. This precarious position can happen whether you are in a nursing home or not. There are thousands, perhaps millions, of older (and younger) persons who simply give up the desire to live simply because no one wishes to take them into account. The fact that suicide is now one of the top ten causes of death would suggest that dying is for many persons preferable to living.

A person once said, "The death of love evokes the love of

death." So true. The degree to which we feel that we belong to somebody or to some group, goes a long way toward explaining our will to live or our will to die. If we sense a relatedness, a sharing of mind, body, and spirit, the desire for continued engagement is strong. But if we feel disconnected and unloved, suicide may emerge as an option.

Sometimes we are so intensely into a relationship we are willing to die for it. That is, feeling that we are a burden, we may wish to spare loved ones the economic, social, and psychological pain of our dying. In this case, we disengage from life *out of love* rather than as a result of the *death of love*.

And finally, for some there may be no perceived relationship in which engagement is possible. A silent roommate, blindness, hearing impairment, stroke, etc., may so devastate a person's social world that he or she loses any thought of ever engaging in a meaningful relationship again. In short, there is no other or group of others with whom sharing is possible. Life is over even though the body may survive.

In each of these cases, a nursing home resident may decide to place his or her dentures on the tray and sneak silently into the next life (whatever that may be). Some have even been successful in having the nasogastric (forced feeding) tube removed so that they could be allowed to die. There will be others.

The importance of relationship is critical to life and living, and it is equally important in terms of death and dying. The most important question we can ask a nursing home resident is, "Who loves you?" As suggested earlier in this book we rarely ask it. All too often we anticipate the person will say, "Nobody loves me," and this to be followed by tears. In brief, we don't ask the question because we are afraid of the answer. And the answer might hurt . . . us!

The entertainer Dean Martin used to sing, "Everybody loves somebody sometime." If a resident has no one who loves him/ her – no aide, no family, no roommate, no housekeeper, no minister, no nurse, no doctor, no guardian, no friend, no one – then we had better organize a love-in before our resident checks out. And if no one can be found, and the resident desires none, we must honor his/her decision to withdraw from life into death.

Anyone reading this book is, in some way, involved in the nursing home drama. As the authors, we believe that each of you, and ourselves, have as our responsibility, the relationship needs of those who live full-time in a home. Fortunately the colony *is* a human one. Everybody does love somebody sometime. In the nursing home where she worked for three years, Sally observed that each resident, no matter how seemingly unappealing or difficult, was some staff member's favorite.

But as in the larger society, relationing can easily change in form and content. And in the nursing home, it changes all the time. There is much turnover among both residents and staff. People die, people get fired, people leave. Becoming membered to another human spirit, and having it last, is often problematic.

As sure as the sun will rise tomorrow, there is someone in every nursing home in America who, although alive, is in desperate need of your love. What a great opportunity this presents. You can go to them and give them a reason for living. You can give them the gift of life itself. And they will return it.

PLAY

The danger in discussing play as a factor in old age is the confronting specter of old age as a "second childhood." The concept of second childhood produces, in its darkest form, these obscene and insulting birthday cards which purport to be humorous about aging. But, we mustn't be scared away by sick jokes when the concept contains the good seed of a better understanding.

In old age, as in childhood, the load of responsibilities is usually minimal. This is particularly true for those who have entered the nursing home. We recall our friend, Arthur, who when confronted with a bill for medical expenses which he couldn't pay, declared with all of the confidence of an 80-year old, "Let them come and get me!" He knew they wouldn't; he also knew they would have if he had been young or middle-aged.

Another nursing home friend, Phyllis, phoned a department store in response to a bill charged in her name. "I live in a nursing home," she announced. "I go to the doctor and the dentist and out to dinner. I do not shop!"

I do not shop, I do not go to work. I do not keep house. I do not own property. I do not drive a car. I do not get meals or call service repair people. I do not mow the lawn. I live in a nursing home.

In the nursing home where she worked, Sally discovered why women who had been renowned cooks and caterers in their day never complained about the food; they were too delighted to have three square meals placed in front of them each day with nothing required of them. An older person in a nursing facility, even as a child in a secure home, has free time. And if one's inclination is like a child's in not requiring much more than a few other people and an active imagination, then free time means that one can play. We recall with pain our own early dignity, reserve, and stiffness that kept us from entering in to the world of the nursing home with a child's sense of fun. But the residents cured us.

Sally remembers a dignified woman whose wheelchair was always placed next to the restroom which Sally used. Every day they nodded formally. Once, however, when Sally was feeling skittish, she said to the woman as she approached to door, "How much do you charge for the use of your toilet?"

"Twenty-five cents on Tuesdays and Thursdays, but you're out of luck—I'm closed today!" Ethel and Sally were free to play together.

What is the nature of elderly play as we understand it? It is not, first of all, the kind of adult play which people move to Sun City and other retirement communities to indulge in. We are talking about something beyond that when physical and sometimes material losses have carried persons into a less active, more circumscribed existence. Here is the time and place to free ourselves from the leftover dregs of our responsibility-burdened middle age and/or the challenges and complacencies of retirement. It seems to us that in frailer old age we need to recapture what we had when we were new at living—spontaneity. We do not, after all, have plans anymore; not the kind of plans we used to have. We are nearer to death than anything else, and each day remaining to us is an entity unto itself.

A friend tells the tale of his grandmother who had assumed a biblically set age limit for herself of fourscore years. Having passed 80 and being still alive, she believed she had "done her duty" and proceeded to take each day as a kind of bonus to be simply and fully enjoyed.

Reflect for a moment on how children play. They leave the house and head out into the neighborhood. They encounter another child and imagination takes over — they play. They may have no physical props at all. Their spontaneity creates and allows it to happen.

The old folks in the nursing home do the same. They leave their rooms and head for the line-up, the lobby, and the busy intersections. They are ready for the encounter that will make the moment. Even if memory has failed, the moment is still there to enjoy. The experience reminds them of their own and another's humanness.

Each age has its advantages and its burdens. Children are unselfconsciously children. Old people need to be unself-consciously old people and to be accepted and enjoyed by others as such. Recapturing the capacity for playfulness then becomes not part of a sick joke, but the return of a precious gift misplaced during the journey.

Have you lost the knack of playing? How spontaneous are you? Are you free to be yourself? Can you allow others to be free?

If we continue to play uncomfortable games of pretense, pray only for our loved ones to be "normal" again, disengage from relationships which were previously meaningful, and refuse to allow ourselves the freedom to laugh and play in the midst of our pain and suffering, then there is no hope. Only in accepting our own vulnerability, indeed, our own finitude, can we begin to accept it in others. We hope the reader has, by now, begun to anticipate and see the nursing home and those who live within it, with new eyes. We hope the human spirit which uniquely characterizes each one of us, and which dwells deep within, is seen as something which is always within reach if we will stop and say, "Hello in there."

Looking beyond wrinkles and a fading memory is, however, a difficult task for persons who have spent much of their lives in the presence of a wholly different personality and spirit. Perhaps this is why it is sometimes a bit easier for a housekeeper or a nurses' aide, who have not been previously intimate with the resident/patient, to love on more unconditional terms. At any rate, we clearly understand how overwhelming the challenge can be. If any hope is to be found, we feel it lies in the ability of each one of us to come to a new understanding about matters of life and death.

Fifty years ago, two desperate men, Bill W. and Dr. Bob, found a stairway which led them out of the pit of alcoholic despair. Having taken their last drinks, these two men stayed sober for the rest of their lives—the one for 37 years, the other for 15.

In the early years of their sobriety, they looked back into the deep place from whence they had come and saw that the steps they had climbed were not random toe-holes, but as in a maze, the only way out of the pit. Thus were born the Twelve Steps, which together with the rest of the Alcoholics Anonymous plan of recovery, has enabled over a million people in some 115 countries to achieve and maintain sobriety.

More than that, the Twelve Steps represent to most AA members an approach to living that has freed them from the burdens of the past, given new meaning to the present, and confidence of the future. Experience has taught that a serious and sincere effort to follow and fulfill these Steps enables the alcoholic to die to the old personality and way of viewing the world, and to be born into a new way of being and understanding life.

These Steps were created out of recovery and inspiration, and tested by the fire of experience. There is nothing casual about them; they are a program, a process. Although they are neither rigid nor neat, as life is neither rigid nor neat, they have, nevertheless, an integrity in their order testified to by those who have journeyed through them. A Step well-taken leads naturally to the next one; a Step skipped may lead to a fall. Some people move through the Steps with fair speed while others may take years. Some go back and redo the steps on a daily basis; others work them periodically. But the key is that when faithfully done, they work.

The genius of AA's Twelve Steps lies in the fact that though the treated illness is alcoholism, the cure requires a transforming change in attitudes, beliefs, and behavior. Because this method has been so successful in healing one disease, the Twelve Steps have been adopted by programs treating narcotics addiction, eating disorders, parenting, sex, and relationship problems—all with positive results. Individuals in the fields of religion and mental health are among the chief advocates of the Twelve Step process, recognizing that the Steps confront basic human life distortions, and offer recovery of the spiritual humanness which is the essence of living.

Looking back over our book, we discovered our own story: we had originally been in a state of denial and unhappiness about aging and death. When we went into nursing homes, our disease became acute, and we descended into a deep hole. But we found a way out—we discovered a new way of living with what had been the twin monsters of aging and death. With different ways of looking, thinking, feeling, and behaving, we found friends where we had once seen only strangers, and gardens where there had once been only pits.

In a moment of inspiration, David realized we had gone through a "Steps" process. If, using that AA formula, we could describe and interpret what we did and how it changed us, our experience could become more than something to share with others—it could become a process, a pattern for people to adopt.

And make no mistake, for most of us human beings, fear and avoidance of aging and death is an illness. It does little good to moralize with people or attempt to inspire them in an effort to promote greater acceptance of and involvement in nursing home life. Sooner or later, guilt and/or high-mindedness will prove inadequate. We have seen too many eager and sincere nursing home volunteers falter and drift away. Training programs for volunteers and support groups for families of residents may create more understanding and buttress the willpower, but they are only creative and symptom treating—not re-creative and healing. We have come to see that unless we offer this Twelve Step process for recovery from the fear and avoidance of the aging and death of ourselves and others, our book will fall into the former category. Our fondest hope is that these Twelve Steps (adapted from Alcoholics Anonymous and modified to meet the needs of persons confronted by aging and death), together with the magic of the residents, will allow healing to happen and love of nursing home life to be born.

TWELVE STEPS TOWARD THE AFFIRMATION OF AGING AND DEATH

1. Admitted we were powerless over the reality of death, and could not control the aging process.

Aging, physiological aging that is, begins in late adolescence and continues until the organism dies. This is true for every living thing, including humans. While there have been some bizarre attempts over the centuries to protect and preserve life at all costs, all living things nevertheless die. Life endures for only a given season, and then it is over.

While we invite the reader to seek his or her own explanation concerning the meaning of death, we are convinced that it is intended. That is, it is part of the Creation. But given the fact that a diversity of opinion abounds on this subject, suffice it to say that while life can be a most wonderful experience, it most certainly ends. And while we may not like it, we have no control over the process. Oh, some may decide to end their lives prematurely, and thereby feel as if they have seized the moment of death for themselves, but that is all they have done. They have only brought about its inevitability sooner than it otherwise would have happened.

Having no control over aging and death, we are indeed powerless to stop it. It is this powerlessness, this helplessness, that drives us insane. As we watch our loved ones die before our eyes, we want to reach out and make them whole again. We want them to be normal forever. Such is the case with doctors, nurses, ministers, guardians, and others as well, but there are no more yesterdays. There is no going back. The key is to learn to accept those we love the way they are rather than the way we want them to be. These steps will help us do this, but we must first admit the reality that none of us gets out of this alive.

With our minds we know that no one gets out of this life alive, but our feelings tell us we will be the exception. The absurdity of it makes no difference. We human beings are so constituted as to be the natural center of the universe, with even grief for loved ones primarily a reflection of our own personal loss.

No doubt this is why dealing with our own aging and death drives us into insidious self-deception and avoidance. Even some who claim a religious faith that covers and undoes the finality of death may be side-stepping death's reality. Whatever happens after death, dying is the final curtain on the self as it has been lived in the flesh. That end of self, which is the only way we have experienced life, is frightening to contemplate, let alone accept. And the aging of the body and the mind are not only facts that must be confronted in themselves, but also neon signs flashing the news that we are on our way out.

It is little wonder that most of us fall prey to some form of fear and denial. Avoiding thoughts of death may be easier if we are fortunate in long-lived family and friends, but personal aging is another game altogether. The unreadable print lets us know that only with the artificial help of glasses will our eyes ever function normally again. Efforts to keep our teeth, our figure, our physical dexterity, our hair, our skin tone, and our memory, become conscious purposes of everyday life. We modify our diet, adopt an exercise program, try new creams, distribute our hair more carefully, floss and brush with new dedication, make lists, and write everything down we need to remember. At its best this can be a positive response and adaptation to aging, but for most of us it also carries an element of avoidance. At its worst, it leads to denial efforts in more extreme forms.

Whatever we do, however we appear, we are still inexorably aging and dying. The real battlefield therefore, is not our bodies, but our minds and feelings. And the necessary act is not one of courage, but of surrender to what will be.

2. Came to believe that we needed to be restored to sanity.

To go on living with the guilt, anxiety, and fear produced by our failure to accept the deteriorating conditions of our loved ones will get us nowhere. The insanity can become so unbearable that we even stop visiting the person for whom we care so much. We may begin our griefwork long before they die, and as a result, have them dead long before they are dead. If we do not come to believe that something can restore us to sanity, there will, in fact, be no hope, no sanity.

In the scheme of things, everything that lives, ages and dies. In that sense I am no different from the slowly crawling fly on the windowsill or the browning leaf on the tree. In due time, the fly will be stilled and the leaf will fall to the ground. I, too, will be stilled and dropped into the earth.

Insanity exists to the degree that I see myself as different and try to perpetuate that difference by deliberation or denial. It may seem innocent enough to avoid thoughts of my own aging and death or to bemoan them. But the minute I disassociate myself from the billions of human beings who have been born, aged, and died, I become self-centered, special, and arrogant. My biggest problem may be that I perceive this worry and avoidance as natural and normal. But, what does it do to me? Let's look at it.

My stomach knots when I pass a cemetery. Attending a funeral takes a real effort of will because I am so uncomfortable in the presence of death. I skip the television programs and don't go to the movies that are about "sad things." I am awkward and ill-at-ease around anyone with a possible terminal diagnosis and feel inadequate in my response to the bereaved. I either put off making a will or do it with much suppressed inner fear. I brush aside my aging parent's attempts to discuss anything connected with his or her death.

All of this began long ago with distress over aging. I was depressed, really depressed, by my 40th birthday, but I never confronted that depression or worked it through. White hairs in my eyebrows or my beard, a newly observed wrinkle, the uncovered gray in the part-line, the crepey skin on my upper arms and thighs, the inability to do something as easily or as well or as fast as I used to do it—any of these factors could ruin a large part of my day. Observing similar signs of aging in friends and those I loved caused fear and anxiety. I intentionally avoided places where the aging and the dying might be congregated. When a loved one or friend moved to a nursing home, I was forced by my own inner turmoil to make an enormous effort of will to visit them or unsatisfying rationalizations for not visiting them.

I was, in short, at odds with my aging self and the certainty of my eventual death. Uncomfortable with self, I could not give genuine comfort or assurance to others: I either avoided and denied or forced myself and suffered.

Isn't this insanity? Isn't it crazy not to be able to live life fully for myself and others because I am denying the basic "okayness" of Creation? When I think of a world in which death didn't exist and face its implications, cannot I get at least a hint of the possible necessity of aging and death? Isn't it insane to continue on in a denying and depressed state when I could be living serenely with my own aging—keeping my touch light and my humor intact? Don't I need to believe that I can be restored to sanity?

3. Made a decision to accept aging and death as a natural part of the Creation.

Whatever or whoever had the power to create the universe — and all the life that dwells within it — must have intended aging and death to be part of the design. And despite our most imaginative efforts to slow the process down, by either denying it or by covering it up in some way, it goes on. Our attempts to intervene do nothing to influence the outcome. Thus, while we may not appreciate the finality of life, we find ourselves in the difficult position of like it or not, it's going to happen. The best alternative is to accept it as a natural part of the Creation. To think otherwise puts us in a no-win situation.

How sad to be so preoccupied with something that is unalterable, and as a result, blind to the special lived·moments, joys, and celebrations that life has given us. We should be grateful, not resentful, of the opportunities that our short life spans have provided.

We have to learn to live in the NOW. Today is the day that counts. As a great philosopher from India once proclaimed, "Yesterday is but a dream, and tomorrow is but a vision, but today, well-lived, makes every yesterday a dream of happiness, and every tomorrow a vision of hope." All we have been given, and all we can be sure of, is today. Live it well and be grateful.

A conscious, intentional decision is the action required of us. We will accept the natural order of the Creation which includes aging and death, and we will assume and affirm its okayness. When our old fears and denials come into our minds, we will reassert our decision to take life as it has been given to us, and trust in its ultimate good. We will make plans based on the reality of the greater plan over which we have no control. We will make a decision to be sane.

4. Made a searching and fearless moral inventory of ourselves.

Everywhere it seems we are bombarded with youth, sex, and fast times in this high tech, rapid moving world of ours. Anything used and obsolete gets discarded — including garbage, old tapes, and aging bodies. Newspapers, magazines, movies, and television shows reveal a social milieu of people on the make, on the rise, and young. Old folks, particularly the confused ones, are shuffled off to the city dump located over the hill or behind the trees. Their place is no longer in the mainstream. Stranded in the overflow puddles, they eventually die belly-up as the current sweeps past.

We fight to stay in the mainstream for the alternative is too horrible to imagine. We certainly don't want to be like them! "Oh God, please keep me out of the nursing home!" we say. The thought of sitting in that line-up with a distinctive yet expressionless face is too much for us. We don't want any part of it. We only see tubes catching our pee and bedpans catching our poop. To us it is like being hooked up to the respirator with no hope of a code blue. That is, even if we want to be disconnected, life goes on. In the nursing home, we see our fate as a living death. We see a leper colony, not a human one.

Our fear and our anxiety and our guilt about growing old and dying a living death are too much for us. And our guilt is intensified ten-fold if we collaborate with other executioners in sentencing one of our loved ones to this fate. Putting them in the very place we dread most causes our guilt to turn to shame, and in turn, our shame to despair. Often we suffer much more than the person we have committed.

How then do we stop our downward plunge from guilt to shame, and to that final despair which we label "resignation?"

In doing the first three Steps, we have placed our feet firmly on the secure path—the one that will get us where we want to go. We have begun to accept the fact of aging and death as normal and natural, as part of the okayness of Creation. In our new mood of acceptance, we are ready to look back at what we did when avoidance and denial were our motivating forces. We are ready for Step Four.

Taking Step Four is rather like going to the dentist to have a particularly bothersome tooth pulled. We have suffered from its dull ache for a long time, but have been content to deal only with its symptoms. We have lessened its ache with patent medicines and avoided icy foods. Anything, we felt, was preferable to the dynamics of the dentist's chair. Better the constant ache of avoidance than the exquisite pain of removal.

But, we have changed. We are now ready to face the moment of pain in order to be free from the continuous ache.

The Fourth Step *is* painful. It is painful because it requires unqualified honesty about our most hidden thoughts and motivations, and a clear-eyed scrutiny of our actions. We will have courage to do this to the degree that we believe it is absolutely necessary to our healing and happiness.

What will we find as we dig into our attitudes and actions? We will certainly discover dozens of ways in which we have covered up and denied our own aging. We will no doubt recall overhearing or reading an objective description of our aging selves that cut us to the quick. Facing this type of self-delusion makes us squirm.

On another level, we may have experienced real resentment toward the person who talked to us about will-making, cemetery plot selection, or the need to make personal funeral arrangements. And remember the person who was so callous as to remark that someone we loved was "failing"? We have avoided and pretended to ourselves so consistently that accuracy and realism strike us as insensitive.

On a practical level, we will recognize that our inability to face the future openly has resulted in our burdening others. A wife may need to admit that her husband is forced to make most of their plans regarding aging and death because she does not like to talk about such things. A widower may come to the painful realization that he kept his wife at home under his own care too long; her comfort and well-being would have been better served elsewhere, but he could not bear to think of her in a nursing home. This is hard stuff—the stuff that makes tears of regret. But we must not avoid it if we are to get well.

We will have to deal with our "visiting failures"—our neglect of real time sharing with the homebound and nursing home elderly in our lives. We need to feel the pain of deep regret that our own self-centered avoidance and denial kept us from sharing the precious gift of ourselves with them.

Some of us will be faced with the need to deal with current problems in a new, self-honest way. Much as I love my mother, am I really prepared to take her into my own home and care for her when the need arises? Being rigidly honest with myself may require me to face limitations in my love. Perhaps my motivations would be more guilt and family pressure than love. Perhaps I am caught up in a need to perceive myself as the devoted child when, in fact, I harbor very mixed feelings toward my parent. It may be that in spite of genuine and deep love, I know I would resent giving up all of the things I would have to give up to fulfill such a role. Whatever my conclusions, a commitment to truth is required.

When we work with ourselves in this manner, we are doing the Fourth Step—we are making a searching and fearless moral inventory of ourselves in relation to aging and death. We may need to write down our inventory as we take it in order to reinforce our musings and to keep an account.

Above all, we must not be afraid for the rewards are great. An honest facing of ourselves is the only way we can prepare to throw off the shackles that have held us prisoner.

5. Admitted to ourselves and to another human being the exact nature of our wrongs.

Aware of our negative and distasteful feelings and attitudes toward aging and death, we need to do more than inventory them for ourselves. We need to share what we have done and how we feel with another human being. Admitting our horror and uncomfortable feelings about the local nursing home and the people who live in it, is necessary. To do otherwise will only enhance personal feelings of guilt and shame, and it will further isolate us from others. It is important that we discover that we are not so unique, not different, just human. Encounters of this kind require a special understanding. Most persons, when confronted with something out of the ordinary, something less than normal, something less than we want it to be, recoil and resist further interaction. The temptation is to avoid it at all costs. If we are unable to confess these basic human tendencies, we may never be at peace with ourselves.

Sharing our fear, pain, and frustration with another person is a liberating experience. All of a sudden we are not alone. Our pain is shared, understood. We can now talk about it. We can begin to get honest.

Trust in the other is, however, a prerequisite for this kind of undertaking. We must be very selective to whom we confess our story. A close friend and confidant is sometimes best. A counselor or minister are good options too. In short, a person with whom we have shared previous secrets, but who nevertheless continues to accept us, is the kind of other we are suggesting here. Complete trust is the key.

We need to receive the same kind of acceptance we are so desperately desiring to give to our loved one in the nursing home. Moreover, if we are able to experience it, we may, by the grace of God, be able to pass it on. Thomas Merton once said, "Divine strength is not usually given us until we are fully aware of our weakness."

6. Were entirely ready to be free of our defects of character.

Sharing character defects is one thing, wanting to be free of them is something else. It is ironic that the way some people talk creates the impression that they actually enjoy dwelling in their self-pity. Whether it is due to a search for sympathy or an acceptance of helplessness, they cry out in despair. To want to be free of this unhappiness would, we think, be natural. But one must be ready.

We must be ready to be relieved of these negative emotions, and we must mean it. So often our cries are for understanding rather than for change. The successful working of this step is to be willing to have our old ways of responding taken from us. Willingness is the key and it is all that is required.

7. Sought humility to replace our shortcomings.

Humility is not a state of mind with which many of us are familiar. We have encountered humiliation a time or two—a terrible experience of self-lowering forced on us from the outside—but humility is different. It is a self-lowering that happens inside ourselves. In its best sense, it suggests that we are in our rightful place in the universe—one among many, sharing the same weaknesses, fears, hopes, shortcomings, and needs as those around us. We acknowledge our interdependence and know that we cannot make it alone. We also accept the fact that what we do or don't do affects those around us for good or ill.

If we have done the previous Steps well and honestly, we will be acutely aware of our own failings. The confrontation with our past and with those parts of our character that have hurt others and harmed ourselves will have left us in a state of genuine humility. Knowing what we are and what we have done in the face of aging and death, we are ready to be rid of our faults and self-deluding habits.

If we are people who believe in God, we will ask for God's help with this. We may, on the other hand, have only a sense of some other source of power in the universe whose force we acknowledge. Whatever our personal beliefs, we will be aware that we are asking for help.

The Seventh Step is the desire and the seeking to have our shortcomings removed. It leads us naturally into the Eighth Step where we must become willing to reach out to others in a genuine effort to heal our own past and theirs.

8. Made a list of all persons we had harmed, and became willing to make amends to them all.

The Twelve Steps are a process that requires us to keep moving forward. We cannot, for example, settle into a state of good feeling which the newfound humility of Step Seven has brought us. There is to be no "general confession" followed by dismissal with a blessing. Instead, we are told in Step Eight to sit down and make a list of all the people we have harmed by our fear and avoidance of aging and death and become willing to put things right with them. This is indeed hard.

We have admitted in the previous Steps that our attitudes and fears about aging and death have caused us to hurt others. Unintentional as it may have been, we must own up to the part we have played in their hurt. Now we are required to name the persons we have harmed with the idea of becoming ready to make amends to them. It is a great leap from the private inventory-taking and sharing with one another of the Fourth and Fifth Steps, to the active amends-making of the Ninth Step. Wisely, we are given this Eighth Step as a bridge and a preparation.

We must sit down and make a list. In doing so we will be confronted by problems and questions which must be worked out. Some of the people we have harmed are dead. This does not let us off the hook; we must be willing to make our amends to them as best we can in the spiritual sense. If we are striving for self-honesty, we will also discover that we have harmed people whom we had not previously counted as among our "victims." Let's take a hypothetical example.

Harry and Anna were our beloved neighbors. Because their only child lived across the country and could visit but once a year, we became Harry's and Anna's mainstay for both practical and emotional support. When they moved to a retirement home, we visited them regularly—until, that is, Anna began to fail. We understand now that the "busyness" that so limited our visits was really an avoidance of the changes in Anna which we didn't want to face. We know we must make spiritual amends to the now deceased Anna.

We need to think carefully about making amends to Harry too. Some might believe that bringing up past hurts to an old man would only hurt him further. On the other hand, our failure to visit Anna, and our failure to share with Harry the pain of her changes and dying, may still be burdening him in a way which we have the power to relieve. We will need to seek humble guidance in deciding which is the best course to take. It is Harry, rather than ourselves, who must be our first consideration.

But, wait a minute. There is a third person in this drama. There is Harry's and Anna's daughter. She confidently believed that we were fulfilling our old role of companion and support to her parents. We recall our guilt when she expressed her deep gratitude to us at Anna's funeral. Admittedly, we have always been a little critical of this woman for not visiting her parents more often. "She could manage if she really wanted to," we used to think. But now that we have taken an honest inventory of ourselves, we are not casting brickbats at anyone. The only point that matters here is that the daughter was misled and we let her parents down. This is the fact which we need to accept. Our evaluation of her character is irrelevant. What is relevant, is whether it would be more hurtful to Harry's and Anna's daughter to disabuse her of her beliefs.

It becomes obvious how much we need this Eighth Step preparation before we begin the Ninth. We need to take the time to think things through thoroughly, to weigh possible actions carefully, and to seek guidance. We must always keep in mind that while amends-making is a vital part of our own healing, it must be responsibly directed for the good of others. An encouraging note: AA members who practice this Step find most amends recipients are amazed and delighted.

9. Made direct amends to such people wherever possible, except when to do so would injure them or others.

One begins to see a pattern in these Steps to Recovery. There is the preparation Step in which we must summon every ounce of honesty and courage to probe deep within ourselves. We must take our motives and actions out of the box where we have hidden them and dust them off. Holding them up to the light, we see them for what they are and become willing to clean them off and let them go.

Notice, however, that an inward Step is always followed by an outward one. Once we have done our homework, we are required to "turn it in." Reflection is followed by action. So, having prepared ourselves in the Eighth Step, in the Ninth we engage others in amends-making.

With as much wisdom as we can command, we have decided to whom we need to make amends. We have given our best thought and sought guidance for those difficult areas where our openness might cause injury or hurt to others. We have undoubtedly made at least one decision to refrain from amends-making for what we believe to be the best interest of other people. Now it becomes a matter of timing with those to whom we must express our sorrow and sadness for what we have done or left undone.

Timing *is* important. We must not rush forward to make amends in a self-centered fashion, eager to get a difficult job behind us. If we do so, we will miss the point. If being truly willing to make amends is our motive, we will be sensitive to the right method and the right moment. If we run into unavoidable delays, we will accept them positively, believing that the moment is not right.

We may make some helpful discoveries. Suppose we have decided to write our amends to someone, but find ourselves tearing up letter after letter, dissatisfied and frustrated. This is the time to take our problem to a trusted friend who understands what we are trying to do. With objective help, we may find that writing a letter was another manifestation of our old fault, avoidance, and that we need to go to the person directly by phone or visit. With all of the self-honesty we have been exercising, we will be able to recognize truth and embrace it gratefully when it appears.

We make amends because we must. If it blesses the lives of others and heals relationships, that is indeed a bonus. If, on the other hand, someone does not understand our amends-making or remains bitter toward us, we must accept it as philosophically as possible, knowing we have done what we had to do.

10. Continued to take personal inventory and when we were wrong promptly admitted it.

Working Steps One through Nine can begin to get us on course, but there is still much work to be done. We have to continually inventory our thoughts, feelings, and actions toward imperfect and dying persons. It is incredibly easy to come up with new excuses for not visiting our friend or relative in the nursing home. And the longer we put if off, the easier it becomes to disengage altogether.

Accepting our loved one in a frail condition as opposed to a normal and healthy one is particularly difficult. After all, we have spent years, very often a lifetime, with our friend or relative under better circumstances. Our memories are filled with laughter, excitement, play, joy, good times, trips, and other special shared moments. To see them now, separated off in a community of companions who share their same misery, is too much for us. We may be able to visit once or twice, but repeated visiting calls us into a commitment for which we are not prepared. This is why the Tenth Step is so important. We must continue to take personal inventory and when we catch ourselves falling back into our old ways of thinking and acting, we must admit it, and deal with it.

Special holidays and anniversaries can be difficult. Christmastime, for example, can evoke all kinds of memories. To celebrate around the tree and to share in a turkey feast knowing that Mother or Grandmother may be eating off a paper plate with a plastic fork, may ruin an otherwise happy time of gladness, peace, and joy.

Fluctuating between these high and low moments can be devastating if we forget to work the steps. We must always be on guard, prepared for the worst. And when our reactions are inappropriate, less accepting and more self-pitying, we must promptly admit it.

A quick recall of our experience with Steps One through Nine will help get us back on track. We must realize that our lives will continue to be unmanageable if we cannot accept the fact that we have absolutely no control over the aging process. There will be no hope, no sanity, until we make a decision to accept aging and death as a natural part of the Creation. Our denial of these realities gets expressed in a number and variety of ways, but it will help if we share our negative thinking and behaving with others. That is, if we want relief, we will get ready to free ourselves of these defects of character, and we will humbly seek to replace our shortcomings. Making a list of persons we have not loved and accepted as they are, and making amends to them (such as making a decision to visit them regularly), will indeed move us from depression and despair to acceptance and hope. And when we begin to fall into our old ways of thinking, we work Step Ten. We continue to take a personal inventory of ourselves, and when we discover we are wrong, we promptly admit it.

11. Sought through reflection and deliberate contact with frail older persons the acceptance of life as it is and the power to live it.

In the Twelve Steps of Alcoholics Anonymous, the Eleventh Step reminds the alcoholic of the importance of improving his or her conscious contact with a Higher Power. It is God, as understood by the alcoholic, that provides the guidance and power with which a person can live successfully; and to stay sober, conscious contact is necessary. In our Twelve Steps Toward the Affirmation of Aging and Death, we have, for reasons cited earlier, minimized the emphasis on God, but we do encourage deliberate contact with frail older persons.

In most instances of prejudice, increased interaction with a negatively stereotyped group decreases prejudice and increases acceptance. This has clearly been our experience with older persons in nursing homes. They have taught us how to live in the midst of a dying community. We have seen, in their lives, the power and strength of the human spirit. And, speaking of Higher Powers, in most cases these wonderfully frail older people tell us that it is their faith in God that pulls them through.

Deliberate and regular visiting in nursing homes can indeed be a liberating experience. The many stories we have shared in this book are repeated all across America—in these total communities, all kinds of humor, love, kindness, patience, understanding, caring, and honesty get played out every day. Episodic, rare, or brief visits will only enhance already negative stereotypes of the setting and the people who live in it. A ritualized and disciplined pattern of visiting, on the other hand, will quickly turn the leper colony into a human one. The regular visitor will discover the beauty and power of old age, not ugliness and decay.

Residents who live in the world of the nursing home have taught us how to live and how to die. Both are done with grace and dignity. Acceptance of our own aging and dying is the gift they have given to us.

12. Having had this awakening as the result of working these steps, we tried to carry this message to others.

The awakening occurs when we come to realize that "normal" means there is a time for living and a time for dying, and that this is true for every living thing. We cannot retard aging and we cannot prevent dying. Doctors, more than any other professional group, need to learn this; the family, more than any other social institution, needs to embrace it too; and every individual, every human being, needs to acknowledge its reality most of all. To be human means to grow old and die. Once accepted, all the other dimensions of humanity can begin to surface in all their splendor.

Once our own finitude and the finality of life in others is acknowledged, we begin to make every day count. We focus on the now, not on yesterday or tomorrow. We begin to see that each moment shared with another human spirit is a gift. Indeed, we discover that we are ones who are blessed by our visit. Ask anyone who works or visits regularly in a nursing home, and they will tell you, "I just love the people I care for. They are wonderful." And they are.

When we learn to accept the frailty and vulnerability of a 90-year-old nursing home resident, who, in the final phase of life is much like the infant in the early phase, we will be on our way. And we will be so excited by our new approach to life and death, we will carry the message to others.

One of the major reasons why Alcoholics Anonymous is the most successful program of recovery for alcoholics is its emphasis on group support. Indeed, it began because two drunks started talking to each other about their disease. The concern, love, and understanding of the other's problem kept them sober. The fellowship has grown from these two, in the early 1930s, to millions in the 1980s. We are not suggesting that our use of these Steps will lead to any kind of movement of this magnitude, but we do sense that it is important that persons racked with negative nursing home experiences and fears, share them with others. Support groups for families, even for staff who work in nursing homes, would make these Steps all the more powerful. Our own sharing of the stories and experiences in this book has been therapeutic to us. We hope the steps we have borrowed here, along with these lived moments, carries a message to you.

APPENDIX

The Twelve Steps of Alcoholics Anonymous

1. We admitted we were powerless over alcohol—that our lives had become unmanageable.
2. Came to believe that a Power greater than ourselves could restore us to sanity.
3. Made a decision to turn our will and our lives over to the care of God *as we understood Him.*
4. Made a searching and fearless moral inventory of ourselves.
5. Admitted to God, to ourselves, and to another human being the exact nature of our wrongs.
6. Were entirely ready to have God remove all these defects of character.

7. Humbly asked Him to remove our shortcomings.
8. Made a list of all persons we had harmed, and became willing to make amends to them all.
9. Made direct amends to such people wherever possible, except when to do so would injure them or others.
10. Continued to take personal inventory and when we were wrong promptly admitted it.
11. Sought through prayer and meditation to improve our conscious contact with God *as we understood Him,* praying only for knowledge of His will for us and the power to carry that out.
12. Having had a spiritual awakening as a result of these steps, we tried to carry this message to alcoholics, and to practice these principles in all our affairs.

The Twelve Steps reprinted for adaptation with the permission of Alcoholics Anonymous World Services, Inc.